Treating the Aching Heart

A Guide to Depression,

Stress, and Heart Disease

Treating the Aching Heart

*A Guide to Depression,
Stress, and Heart Disease*

Lawson R. Wulsin, MD

Vanderbilt University Press • Nashville

11 10 09 08 07   1 2 3 4 5

Printed on acid-free paper made from
50% post-consumer recycled paper.
Manufactured in the United States of America

This book is the recipient of the 2005 Norman L. and Roselea J. Goldberg
Prize from Vanderbilt University Press for the best project in the area of
medicine.

Library of Congress Cataloging-in-Publication Data
Wulsin, Lawson R.
Treating the aching heart : a guide to depression, stress, and heart disease /
Lawson R. Wulsin.—1st ed.
p. cm.
Includes bibliographical references and index.
ISBN-13: 978-0-8265-1560-5 (cloth : alk. paper)
ISBN-13: 978-0-8265-1561-2 (pbk. : alk. paper)
1. Heart—Diseases—Psychological aspects—Popular works.
2. Depression, Mental—Popular works.
3. Stress (Psychology)—Popular works.   I. Title.
RC682.W85 2007
616.1′20019—dc22
2006038899

CONTENTS

CLINICAL TIPS

ACKNOWLEDGMENTS

My thanks begin where this book began, in the two writing groups that I have attended monthly while working on this book over the past four years. For their help with the proposal, the chapter-by-chapter manuscript revisions, and the never-give-up process of finding the book's way into print, I thank Mary Tom Watts, Judy DaPolito, Mary Ann Schenk, Libby McCord, Greta Holt, Sandy Love, Dave Gressel, Georgia Court, John Court, Joel Singerman, Jane Heimlich, Fedor Hagenauer, Susan Wheatley, and Jocko Magro.

For believing in the book, for representing it for more than two years, and for her editorial and publishing advice along the way, thanks to Vicky Bijur and the Vicky Bijur Literary Agency.

For salary support and departmental resources, thanks to the chairs of my two departments at the University of Cincinnati during the writing of this book—Randy Hillard of the Department of Psychiatry and Jeff Susman of the Department of Family Medicine.

For taking me in during a six-month special academic leave in 2002–2003 to start this book, for giving me an office and their time, advice, revisions, institutional resources, and friendship, I want to thank the members of the Behavioral Medicine Scientific Research Group in the Division of Epidemiology and Clinical Applications of the National Heart, Lung, and Blood Institute, Bethesda, Maryland: Peter Kaufmann, Susan Czajkowski, Jared Jobe, and Mary Jo Smith.

To my friends and colleagues at the American Psychosomatic Society and the Academy of Psychosomatic Medicine I owe much of what I've learned about depression and heart disease.

I have no financial interest in any of the treatments discussed in this book.

Thanks to Cindy Clark, librarian at the NIH Library, for her help with various literature searches; to Jan Warren, medical illustrator in the Department of Surgery, Cincinnati Childrens' Hospital, for illustrating the text; to Kaneto Fukuhara, senior medical graphic designer at the University of Cincinnati, for polishing the figures; and to Dan Davenport, senior medical photographer for the Academic Health Center for Public Relations, University of Cincinnati, for the jacket photo—many thanks.

Thanks to Iris Csik for her contribution of the cognitive therapy case summarized in Appendix I.

For reviewing and revising drafts of the manuscript, thanks to John Beardsley, Susan Boydston, Polly Cherner, Jim DeBrosse, Jerry Fleg, Noel Free, Greg Fricchione, Sarah Goodwin, Loring Ingraham, David Spence, and Victoria Wells Wulsin.

Thanks to Michael Ames and the staff of Vanderbilt University Press for their attentive guidance through the publishing process.

Thanks to Vic and our sons for the time they gave me to work on this book.

And finally, my thanks to the fifteen people who agreed to lend disguised versions of their stories to this book, bringing science to life for me and, hopefully, for you.

Treating the Aching Heart

A Guide to Depression,
Stress, and Heart Disease

CHAPTER 1

The Aching Heart

Gladness of the heart is the life of a man,
and the joyfulness of a man prolongeth his days.
  —Ecclesiastes 30:22

I have full cause of weeping, but this heart
Shall break into a thousand flaws
Or e'er I'll weep. O fool! I shall go mad.
  —Shakespeare, *King Lear*

Paula Volk, sixty-two, spends most of her time in the front bedroom of her two-bedroom house near the flood plains of the Ohio River, watching the clock, as she says. Her father died at sixty-two from his second heart attack. Her mother died at sixty-two of a stroke. For eight years Paula Volk's heart has been troubling her with chest pains, shortness of breath, and exhaustion. She's sick enough now to need a heart transplant, but too sick to be eligible for the operation. How did she, the daughter of a nurse and an engineer, come to this?

Her mother ate too much, drank too much, and spent too much time in bed with depression, Paula says. Determined to defy her mother's genes and her example, Paula skipped the booze and worked hard as a social worker and later as the owner of a small courier business. Aside from carrying some extra weight most of her adult life (usually weighing about two hundred pounds), Paula felt pretty good and considered herself pretty healthy. She smoked a couple of packs a day for forty years and quit in the spring of 1995, when she was fifty-five and the chest pains began. Within the year she developed congestive heart failure and (like her father) diabetes. And then she had a coronary bypass operation. After the operation

1

she slid into a funk, stopped taking care of her house, kept to her bed, and ruminated about suicide day after day.

For most of the next eight years she remained depressed and disabled, untreated for anxiety or depression in spite of frequent treatments for her heart disease.

Seven years after the bypass operation, she agreed to let her family doctor start her on twenty milligrams of citalopram, or Celexa, an antidepressant. It has helped some, but she has remained at the original dose and has had no other treatment. Is it too little too late? When I asked her how much of the last seven years she's spent depressed, she said, "Eighty-five percent." I looked to her husband and he agreed, "Eighty five to ninety percent." She said, "Without my daughter and my husband I'd be dead. I've leaned on him. He's been my Rock of Gibraltar. Her too." There's still love in that tired heart.

On top of her family history of heart attacks, diabetes, and a fatal stroke, Paula Volk's heart disease was the product of at least four major risk factors—obesity, smoking, abnormal lipids, and physical inactivity. It's also likely that she inherited from her mother a vulnerability to depression, which didn't show up until after her first heart attack. But once the depression descended on her seven years ago, it never fully lifted and has gradually grown worse, along with her heart disease. Now she's still here, holding on, hoping for a way to break out.

Over the last fifty years of unprecedented scientific and public health efforts focused on the heart-disease epidemic in the United States and Western Europe, we have come a long way in predicting who might get a heart attack and treating those who do. We've reduced the death rates from heart disease in men, but we haven't reduced the number of people who get heart disease. Heart disease will still kill one out of three of us. And our best models of prediction still miss half the heart attacks. That is, half of all lethal heart attacks in the United States happen to people who didn't know they had heart disease. The established major risk factors for coronary disease don't tell the whole story—not by a long shot, even if we're looking for warning signs.[1] Who makes up this other half, the half that has defied prediction? There's still much we need to know.

For the past fifteen years I've been doing research on, teaching about, and taking care of people with various forms of stress, depression, and heart disease in my job as a professor of psychiatry and family medicine at the University of Cincinnati. Though high blood pressure and mild forms of depression run in my family, when I began this book I'd made it through fifty-plus years with no heart disease that I knew of and only a bout of dysthymia (mild depression over several years) in my early forties. But I knew my turn could come. My chances of experiencing both disorders would only increase with age.

In addition to my interest in my own survival, I'm attracted to the grim pairing of depression and heart disease because they both affect such a large proportion of the population (one in five U.S. citizens will experience a major depressive episode and one in three will die by heart disease); because each disorder by itself inflicts such impressive damage (depression is the illness most likely to disable us and heart disease is the illness most likely to kill us); and because our current understanding of the interaction between the two disorders represents the best story we have about how troubles with the mind, such as depression, contribute over many years to troubles with the body, such as coronary disease, sometimes with devastating but preventable results.

What makes this pair of problems irresistible for any mental health clinician who spends a lot of time in primary care settings is that early recognition and treatment of both disorders in a single person can have such broad healing effects on the patient and the family, reducing grief and suffering not only for the affected person, but also potentially across several generations. To unwittingly ignore this vicious cycle is to court frustration, prolonged heartache, and early death. To break the cycle is gratifying beyond words.

What more do we need to know? Our best models for predicting risk of heart attack come mostly from research on white men. We do less well predicting with women and nonwhite ethnic populations because relatively little good research has focused on problems specific to heart disease in these groups. Women tend to be diagnosed with coronary disease ten to fifteen years later than do men, and when women have heart attacks, they die at twice the rate of men with heart attacks.[2] Why do women have more trouble with heart disease? What do we need to know about women and heart disease to treat them as effectively as we treat men? Good research on these questions has just begun to find its way into print.

We also don't know enough yet about the brain's role in heart disease. There's every reason to expect that the most important pieces of the unfinished heart-disease puzzle will feature the heart's connection to the brain and the central nervous system. It makes good sense that the brain should have a powerful effect on the heart, both in health and in disease. For a long time it has made good sense to patients, doctors, and poets, but people who do research on the brain don't generally talk much with people who do research on the heart. At the world's leading medical research organization, the National Institutes of Health (NIH) in Maryland, the institute responsible for heart-disease research, the National Heart, Lung, and Blood Institute, has never collaborated on a major initiative with the institute responsible for research on mental illness, the National Institute of Mental Health. This organizational equivalent of quarantining the head from the heart is no longer tenable or tolerable, given what we know about the links between the mind, the brain, and the heart. If the NIH can foster ground-breaking initiatives that link disorders of the heart with the kidney or disorders of the heart with strokes, the NIH could, with a hefty dose of political will, foster ground-breaking research on the links between disorders of the heart and of the mind, such as coronary artery disease and depression.

The enormous pharmaceutical research industry has maintained the same turf divisions between the heart and the brain, intentionally avoiding studies of patients who have problems with both organs. The result is that we know much less than we ought to and need to about how treatments for the central nervous system and the cardiovascular system work with each other, and sometimes against each other. The broad sweep of the public health assault on heart disease in the last half of the twentieth century essentially ignored the effects of the mind and the brain on the heart-disease epidemic.

The costs of overlooking the interactions between stress and depression, on the one hand, and heart disease, on the other, have been sizable. And these costs will rise in the near future unless we improve our ability to prevent heart disease and reduce the rise in depression rates. Depression more than triples the chances that a person with a heart attack will die within the next six months, and yet few coronary care units or cardiologists screen for depression following a heart attack. Less than half of all patients with depression and heart disease get effective treatment for the depression. The reasons for this neglect include the traditionally narrow definition of the cardiologist's turf, which for many has not included assessing or treating depression. It's time to change that.

Depression also triples the chances that a person with a chronic physical illness will fail to stick to a chronic illness treatment regimen over three months. Since only about a half of all people with depression get any treatment and only about a fifth get effective treatment, untreated depression often sabotages the management of chronic physical illnesses like heart disease.[3] Patients and the primary care clinicians who help them manage chronic illnesses over many years need effective strategies for preventing depression from undermining their best efforts. Mental health clinicians, most of whom avoid working in primary care settings or on medical issues, often overlook the cardiac risk factors in their depressed patients. Under the cloak of confidentiality we communicate too little with our medical collaborators, who have often perceived us as unavailable or working in a wholly different health-care delivery system. It is time to change that, and there's good reason to believe that, slowly, change is coming. This book aims to help shift that process of change into a higher gear.

D id depression kill my father?" Tom Geraci, seventy, asked me, and then answered his own question. "I think so, coming on top of his heart disease.... He died almost fifty years ago, but I remember those three months leading up to his death more vividly than yesterday."

Tom Geraci is now four years older than his father was when he died, but Tom hardly looks his age. He stands tall and gestures energetically, speaking at a lively clip in his easy professorial baritone. Like his father, Tom has heart disease, but at seventy he walks four miles a day and works full-time, teaching, writing, and running a prominent Jesuit press in the Midwest. He has no intention of retiring for several years—"I have at least two more big projects to tackle." He exudes that biblical "gladness of the heart." On this day he wanted to talk to me about his experience with heart disease.

My father had had a bad heart for some seven or eight years when I was in high school and college. He'd had several heart attacks before the final one, but it was the death of my mother that brought him down, fast. She drowned on a Tuesday afternoon while swimming in the ocean off the coast of Georgia—she was a strong swimmer, swam there every day, often alone. "There was nothing unusual," [my father] said to me, "but she drowned." That was April of 1956, and my father died that July, just three months later . . . and only five days after our wedding.

In 1956, life was tougher for people with heart disease than it is today. Tom's father's was treated with rest and nitroglycerine pills for chest pains for most of eight years. Heart surgery would not become an option for another twenty years. Blood-pressure medications were crude and ineffective by today's standards. Links to cholesterol, physical inactivity, and smoking were just beginning to merit scientific investigation.

Life was even tougher then for people with severe depression. Antidepressant medications didn't exist, and psychotherapy was a cumbersome process better suited for the worried well who could visit an analyst four or five times a week for many months. For Tom's father half a century ago, even good doctors could do little to treat the combination of depression and heart disease. But the story of Tom's father presents the premise of this book: Depression aggravates heart disease, and heart disease aggravates depression. And Tom himself stands for the main message of the book: We can break the cycle of depression and heart disease.

It was no coincidence that he held on until his last child had married, because after my mother died, it took all he had just to hold on. He immediately became paralyzed, not physically but mentally a basket case. He rarely did anything, ate anything, went anywhere. I moved home for the last months of my senior year at Brown University to take care of him, and I watched this highly successful insurance lawyer turn incompetent overnight. He'd fall into fits of tears and long spells of being mute. He hardly saw or talked to anyone but me. Sometimes we had long conversations and he told me that behind his spells of muteness was grief, always about my mother. But this was more than grief. It felt to me at times like he was in a hopeless state of near-death.

As with King Lear, despair took Tom's father beyond common grief to an early death.

For thirty-six of their forty years together my parents had a solid, affectionate marriage, but when I went off to college my mother started drinking. She drank because she was depressed and she was depressed because she drank. He refused to do anything about her drinking. He just gave up. I can't imagine how they communicated during those years. She stopped communicating with me too. The long wonderful talks when I'd come home from school never happened again. So in a way, even before she drowned he'd lost her to depression and drinking—we all had lost her. Those last years were hard on his heart, but those last three months were the hardest.

In the office next to Tom's at the press, his wife Amy now works on the press's special projects. They've shared this work for the last seven years, and they've been married forty-seven years. She too looks younger than her age. "We've had an extraordinary marriage," Tom told me. "I'm more in love with her now than ever."

He told me about the deaths of his parents and the toughest losses of his life with remarkable ease. I wondered about this, and he told me that during divinity school and his early years as a professor of theology he wrote a lot about death. "I've written more about the death of my parents than about anything else." In fact, he wrote a book on Christian approaches to death as a path to resurrection. Soon after its publication, during a routine physical exam in 1985 at the age of fifty-two, he discovered that his high blood pressure, his being fifty pounds overweight, his thirty years of smoking, and his aversion to exercise had put him on a course to match his father's development of heart disease in his fifties. Stunned into action, he quit smoking, started walking four miles a day, and began a medication for his high blood pressure. Several years later he woke up to the realization that alcohol depressed him, and he quit drinking. He immersed himself in daily prayer.

By the time Tom Geraci had that alarming physical exam in 1985, modern medicine had lots to say to him about preventing heart disease, guidance that it had not been able to give to his father. Tom benefited from one of the great public health triumphs of the twentieth century in the United States, the understanding of the heart-disease epidemic and how to treat it. And Tom took the advice of his physician in earnest, behaving like a model patient.

After nine years on this diligent regimen to prevent heart disease, one Wednesday morning in 1994 toward the end of his four-mile walk,

Tom felt dizzy and disoriented and stumbled into a bench. He hurried unsteadily across the lawn to his house, rushed in through the kitchen door calling to his wife, and collapsed on the couch. Evaluation at the emergency department showed that his right carotid artery was severely narrowed, and a later appointment with a cardiologist showed that one of his coronary arteries was also blocked. To prevent a stroke or heart attack, surgery would be required: an endarterectomy to open the flow from his right carotid artery to his brain and a bypass graft around the blocked coronary artery.

Had all those miles Tom had walked done nothing to reduce his risk? Was this bad luck or bad genes making a mockery of his hard work? Had he given up the delightful vices of drinking and smoking only to be stricken with heart disease anyway? Tom didn't see it that way. He put out the call and in the weeks leading up to his surgery received, he said, three hundred letters from family and friends. Some well-wishers warned him to expect pain in his chest wall where the surgeons would crack his sternum and, of course, the depression that commonly follows bypass heart surgery. But he had other plans.

> I don't understand how heart surgery could lead to depression. When I woke up, I was elated. No pain. I was so excited, my blood pressure on the monitor was 205 over 102, dangerously high. I knew I'd better calm down. By then I had learned I could lower my blood pressure by prayer, so I prayed it down. I was fine. The sense of precisely just how fine I was did not leave me. The life that had been almost taken from me had been given back to me.

Call it faith, call it optimism, call it hard-knocks knowledge, confidence, or defiance. Tom Geraci had what it took to sail through heart surgery without capsizing. In fact, he has made it through a long life without suffering the severe depressions that have afflicted his father, mother, sister, and daughter.

> I've hardly lived a life that is depression free, as my wife will tell you, but for the past seventeen years exercise has been my antidepressant. If I go two days without my walks, I'm no good at the office and my wife can tell right away. Like my mother, alcohol depressed me, so I stopped. And prayer helps, so I immerse myself in prayer.

In the eight years since his surgery Tom Geraci has had no symptoms of heart disease. His regimen of two pills for his blood pressure, two for his cholesterol, and an aspirin a day have kept the cardiologist away. He has beaten the odds. The joyfulness of this man "prolongeth his days."

Clinical Tip 1.1: Make use of your family history. Depression and heart disease tend to run in families, for both genetic and environmental reasons, so review with your primary care doctor your family history of heart disease and of depression. Draw a family tree and count the number of close relatives within two generations of you who have had either problem. Making sense of a family history can be complicated, so do it with your doctor. But taking stock of close family members who faced either of these problems, or both, may clarify for you, as it did for Tom Geraci, whether you need to take action and what kind.

Unfortunately, Tom is the exception, not the rule. Good medical advice, lots of work, and timely surgery helped this educated white male narrowly escape the ravages of a stroke or a heart attack, but most people aren't so lucky or so knowledgeable. What about the rest of us, who may not be on such friendly terms with death, depression, and heart disease? And who may have less experience, discipline, luck, faith, or access to good treatment than Tom Geraci had? We will suffer more, get less good treatment, and die younger.

Most of us have not yet benefited from recent scientific advances in this area because of the time gap between scientific advances and their later translation into improvements in clinical practice. This gap, which experts call the innovation diffusion gap, affects all areas of clinical medicine, but it's particularly striking in areas related to neuroscience, which came late to the table. The emergence of sophisticated neuroscience research has lagged a decade or two behind cardiovascular research. Techniques for studying large numbers of brain neurons developed only in the 1980s, and brain imaging didn't achieve a sophisticated state until the 1990s. Consequently, the 1990s was truly the decade of the brain at the National Institutes of Health and around the scientific world. Neuroscience research is now fully dressed, at the table, ready to work. Finally now, the brain researchers and the heart researchers can start talking to each other about the important questions at all levels in ways that translate into better treatment for patients and their doctors.

Consider the questions that remain for research to answer. Is stress sometimes good for your heart? If stress is bad, what kind of stress is bad and for how long? How does depression make heart disease worse? How can grief, misery, or fear put an ache in your heart? Under what conditions can the mind damage the body? What are the biological and behavioral mechanisms by which depression can worsen heart disease? And how does heart disease trigger depression?

These are compelling questions for anyone with depression or heart disease in their family. They are also compelling questions for public health policy makers, because heart disease is the most lethal condition worldwide and depression is the most disabling condition worldwide.[4] These two common and costly conditions often strike the same person, often in ways that escape recognition or treatment, often with devastating but preventable consequences.

The preacher who wrote Ecclesiastes knew about this link. Hippocrates and Shakespeare knew about this link. But in spite of thousands of years of folk wisdom that link despair to the heart, only in the last fifteen to twenty years has good scientific inquiry begun to describe the relationship between these two complex disorders. The aching heart, we now know, is a metaphor rooted in the anatomical links between the neural circuits for chest pain and the neural circuits for emotional pain. A small group of clinical researchers has learned a lot about these links in a short time, but the benefits of this exciting research still have not begun to find their way to the people who most need to know about them—patients, their families, and their doctors.

Scientific advances have a way of hiding in pockets. Even a practical scientific advance does not by itself go where it is most needed. Innovations require translation, packaging, and promotion to reach the people who are most likely to implement or benefit from the advance. In this book you will find the latest scientific thinking on depression and heart disease. Chapter 2 will persuade you that depression is common in people with heart disease, and heart disease is common in people with depression, describing who these people are and the size of this public health problem for our country. This book will change the way you think about depression in

Chapters 3 and 4, the way you think about heart disease in Chapter 5, and the way you think about how these two problems aggravate each other in Chapter 6.

As in Clinical Tip 1.1, I will step aside from time to time to add a clinical suggestion for patients and their doctors. Fascinating stories and enticing scientific facts have a tendency to hang in the air, not quite landing in the realm of practical action. A good test of the clinical value of a story or a fact lies in how readily it translates into a useful clinical application, something you can do. Some of the Clinical Tips presented in these chapters focus on what patients can do; others focus more on what clinicians can do. We will come back in Chapter 9 to the points they raise, elaborating on each and tying them together into a coherent set of treatment strategies. Together these Clinical Tips amount to a collection of suggestions about the current best practices for recognizing and treating depression and heart disease. They do not amount to a treatment plan for any one person. At best they can prompt patients and clinicians to talk more specifically about how to make an individual treatment plan most effective.

The final chapter takes a broad look at the public health dimensions of depression and heart disease. It presents seven strategies for changing our health-care system to improve the treatment of depression and heart disease. And it summarizes what we know and what we still need to learn about this problem.

"Stress" is a broad, inclusive term, free of the stigma of mental pathology. We look at stress the same way we look at bad weather: We expect to have to deal with it. Some forms of stress, like dancing and jogging, are good for the heart. Some forms of stress, usually the chronic or intermittent kinds, are particularly bad for the heart, such as poverty, physical or emotional abuse, and depression. Persistent distress of any kind wears hard on the heart, but so far the scientific evidence for depression's effects on heart disease is more robust than the evidence for other forms of distress. In this book the spotlight follows depression with the understanding that the related forms of distress in the surrounding shadows collaborate on the damage. As we clarify the role of depression in heart disease, we will better understand the roles of the other forms of distress.

The terms "depression" and "heart disease," discussed in detail in Chapters 3 and 5, also require some early clarification. Though both may be defined broadly and used loosely, I will use them in their most important clinical definitions. "Depression" can imply a sad feeling, but I will usually use the term to mean the more enduring and disabling forms of clinical depression, such as major depression, dysthymia, or bipolar depression. The term "heart disease" is a convenient catch-all phrase for at least seven common diseases of the cardiovascular system, some of which don't strictly involve pathology of the heart (such as high blood pressure). The most common and important of these for our public health and for links to depression is coronary disease (also called atherosclerotic heart disease or ischemic heart disease). Other less common forms of heart disease include congestive heart failure, arrhythmias, rheumatic heart disease, and stroke.

For too long the general wisdom about heart disease has ignored the effects of the mind and the brain on the cardiovascular system. The rationale that the brain is too complex to understand scientifically no longer holds water. The brain is now the frontier of modern medicine, the last but most important organ system to be explored. Though we certainly don't understand all we need to know about the brain, we now know enough to sketch the anatomical, physiological, and biochemical links between the brain and the heart.

And for too long the general wisdom about depression has ignored its effects on the rest of the body. For most of the twentieth century, depression was considered primarily a psychological problem, a disorder of mood. We had little idea how profoundly depression disrupts the cardiovascular, the endocrine, and the immune systems, to say nothing of the central nervous system. We now know more specifically how a nervous breakdown ripples through the body and how to treat it.

In spite of the triumph of the public health approach to heart disease, and in spite of great strides in the treatment of mental illnesses with medications and psychotherapy over the last twenty years, the problem of depression and heart disease persists, affecting at least three million adults in the United States every year. One in five people who have a heart attack has major depression, but fewer than half of them get any treatment for depression. If they do get treatment, more often than not it is insufficient. This is true even though depression makes existing coronary disease worse and triples the risk of death within six months of the heart attack. Among the lucky few with coexisting depression and heart disease who get any treatment for depression, less than a quarter get effective antidepressant treatment.[5]

Now that we have learned how to care for the Tom Geracis, we must learn how to care for the Paula Volks of our world. We must learn how heart disease in women, blacks, Hispanics, and Native Americans differs from heart disease in white men. We must learn how to change risky behaviors like smoking and overeating more effectively than we do. We must learn to recognize depression early in the context of the symptoms of heart disease and treat depression aggressively with methods that are safe for the ailing heart. We must identify the people with heart disease whose personal or family histories of depression make them susceptible to depression and try to prevent depression from developing as a complication of heart disease. We must understand how the cycle works in people like Paula Volk— how the biology of heart disease triggers the psychology of depression, which triggers the sociology of poverty and isolation, raising the toll on the already aching heart.

Clinical Tip 1.2: When heart disease strikes, check for depression. Six years of persistent depression passed before Paula Volk started her first treatment for depression. Six years is the average length of time in our country between first symptoms of a mental illness and first treatment, and that is way too long. Getting help doesn't have to take six years. Informed patients and clinicians can beat this common tendency not to recognize depression in the context of heart disease by systematically evaluating depressive symptoms in everyone who develops a major heart-disease event, such as a heart attack or a bypass operation or angioplasty. Identify previous episodes of depression too. For a simple and useful method of measuring depressive symptoms, see the PHQ-9 self-report questionnaire in Appendix D, "Assessment of Depression."

To improve our care, we'll need new ways of thinking about heart disease and new ways of thinking about depression. The old model of heart disease as a plumbing problem is not good enough for Paula Volk. And the old model of depression as an internal conflict over loss or as a disorder of mood is not good enough either. Instead we have to understand that the depression that exerts an influence on heart disease is a disease of the mind, brain, and body. It dramatically and measurably dysregulates (a) stress hormones, (b) the parts of the brain that handle emotions, and (c) the autonomic nervous system throughout the body (the part of the nervous system that automatically regulates basic functions like heart rate and breathing). At the same time, a new model of atherosclerotic heart disease has overtaken the older model, asserting that this form of heart disease is an inflammatory process, in part driven over many years by the same dysregulation of hormones and the autonomic nervous system that is characteristic of depression.

The result of these shifts in the understanding of depression on the one hand and atherosclerotic heart disease on the other is that it is now possible to trace the pathways that link these two disorders. Figure 1.1 shows the major pathways, and Chapter 6 discusses these pathways in detail because they hold the clues for developing more effective strategies to manage depression and heart disease, not just for researchers but also for patients working with their doctors.

Pathway 1 is a behavioral one, which proposes that depression triggers risky behaviors, such as smoking, overeating, and avoiding physical activity, behaviors that raise the chances of developing heart disease or that make existing heart disease worse. Pathway 2 is more directly biological. It proposes that specific biological changes during depression directly accelerate the process of developing heart disease, including elevated stress hormones, changes in heart-rate variability, impaired immune system functioning, and changes in the blood's tendency to clot. In addition, depression may exacerbate other forms of distress (pathway 3), such as chronic anxiety, to overwhelm the central nervous system and then the cardiovascular system.[6]

A word of caution about cause and effect in complex illnesses may prevent misreadings of Figure 1.1 and misunderstandings of the central message of this book, as depicted in the figures in Chapter 7. Complex chronic illnesses such as major depression and atherosclerotic heart disease defy the simple cause-and-effect explanations commonly applied to simpler acute conditions, such as a strep throat infection or food poisoning. Complex chronic illnesses result from the interactions over many years of many factors, some major and some minor, some predisposing to and others exacer-

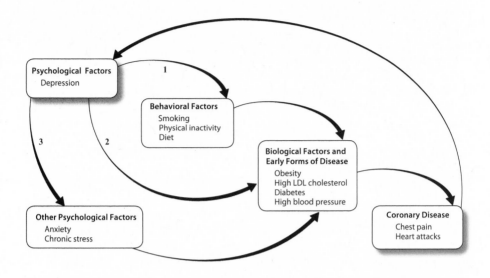

Figure 1.1. Selected Pathways Linking Depression and Heart Disease

bating the development of the illness. Figure 1.1 does not intend to imply that depression is the first or the most important factor contributing to coronary disease. Timing and relative importance of risk factors vary from person to person and from time to time during the course of the illness. Figure 1.1 simply shows the relationship between depression and the other contributing factors along several pathways to the development of heart disease.

These pathways may also work in reverse, as Paula Volk's story suggests. Her first heart attack preceded her first depression. When heart disease strikes first, the demands of the heart disease may overwhelm the mind, leading to depression in a person who has never before been troubled by depression. One way heart disease may trigger depression is by decreasing the blood flow through hardened and narrowed arteries of the brain, specifically those that feed the areas of the emotional brain responsible for mood regulation. The same process that narrows the arteries of the heart often narrows the arteries of the brain. The decreased blood flow may lead to decreased activity in specific areas of the brain in patterns that contribute to severe depression, as described in Chapter 8. When these pathways work in both directions, the elements of a vicious cycle lock into place, driving the person into a downward spiral that is tough to pull out of. For Tom Geraci's father the spiral was lethal, but Tom himself has managed never to get sucked in. For Paula Volk it remains unclear if she will be able to break out.[7]

Is depression a risk factor for coronary disease? Certainly. Is depression a *major* risk factor on the order of smoking, high blood pressure, and obesity? Quite possibly, though important research on this question remains to be done. The current debate about the relative importance of depression among the many factors that contribute to heart disease—even "living in New York City" has been accused of playing a role in heart-disease mortality![8]—will influence some critical scenarios: (a) how much emphasis doctors place on identifying and treating depression in patients with heart disease, and on improving the treatment of heart disease in patients with depression; (b) how much organizations like the American Heart Association and the American Psychiatric Association educate the public about the interactions between depression and heart disease; and (c) whether sufficient money goes into research to answer the remaining questions. This book argues the need for new, large-scale initiatives in all three areas.

Why bother? Why should our health-care system pour precious resources into the problem of depression and heart disease? Some experts have argued that we already know enough about the major risk factors for heart disease and we do not need to look for new ones. We should spend our research efforts figuring out how to change high-risk behaviors in individuals and studying the social and economic determinants of heart disease.[9] I argue that depression worsens most of the risk factors for heart disease and that this fact helps us understand in part why we have such trouble reducing our high-risk behaviors, such as smoking, physical inactivity, and high-fat diets.

Our health-care system should invest its resources in understanding depression and heart disease not only because these are two common, costly, and treatable disorders, but also because the real problem is bigger than these two disorders. The problem we need to understand is how mental disorders contribute to chronic illnesses, and vice versa. Many people with one chronic illness have another chronic physical or mental illness as well. How does depression lead to obesity? How does chronic anxiety fuel chronic pain? How does diabetes add to the risk for depression? How does substance abuse drive the hepatitis C epidemic? How does chronic distress of any kind facilitate the emergence of cancer and interfere with recovery?

For many acute illnesses we now have effective treatments. Our public health priorities are shifting to managing chronic illness, which levies a greater burden on society. The co-occurrence of chronic mental and physical illnesses is a common and costly problem that increasingly consumes larger portions of our health-care budget, now that we have effective treatments for many acute illnesses. We don't yet understand these chronic illness interactions well enough to design effective treatments that break these cycles of influence. A single chronic illness such as heart disease has proven remarkably difficult to understand after half a century at the top of the public health priority list. To understand how two complex chronic illnesses, such as heart disease and depression, operate on each other stretches the limits of the modern medical mind. But that's where the medical mind must go. And we might as well start with depression and heart disease, because we know more about the links between these two than we do about any other pair of mental and physical illnesses.

Does depression's role as a risk factor for heart disease mean that antidepressants could provide a cure for heart disease? No. Just as there's no single cause of any heart disease, there will never be a single medication that can cure or prevent heart disease. Cholesterol-lowering drugs by themselves can't do it. Blood-pressure medications by themselves can't do it. Exercise alone can't do it. Tom Geraci took blood-pressure medications, quit smoking, and exercised daily for ten years, and he still developed heart disease. Too many factors conspire to drive the atherosclerotic heart-disease process over too many years for any one treatment to prevent or cure the disease. Combinations of treatments are essential to prevention and management of most chronic conditions. So the treatment of depression will never by itself be enough, but for people with repeated episodes of depression and for people who experience depression soon after a heart attack, effective treatment of depression may be a lifesaver.

Chapter 9 spells out the lessons for treatment of both heart disease and depression that follow from what we know of the relationship between them. The good news is that depression is treatable and preventable, even when you have heart disease, and that good treatment for depression is good for heart disease. We do not yet know definitively if good treatment for heart disease specifically reduces the risk for depression, but what's good for the heart is good for the mind and the brain. Joy, fish oil, and moderate exercise are all good for the atherosclerotic heart and the depressed mind.

To build a compelling argument for a new approach to these two illnesses, we begin by asking who gets depression and heart disease. Who is at risk and who among us should care enough to change our behavior and our biology to break this cycle?

CHAPTER 2

The Size of the Problem

In 1973, just before my junior year of college, while trying to decide whether to join the then-fashionable rush into medicine, I read a book called *The Body Has a Head*. As much as any book could, this one seduced me into medical school. It's a 784-page dramatist's tour of human physiology by Gustav Eckstein, a retired physiology professor and widely published author at the time the book came out in 1969, when he was almost eighty. Later I met Dr Eckstein, a passionate man, five feet four and a hundred pounds, too small to enlist in the army in World War I. He wore long scarves, even in summer, and glasses with round lenses no bigger than quarters. Though he was a notoriously inefficient teacher of physiology, Eckstein drew crowds of admirers to his lectures at the University of Cincinnati because he performed—always dramatic, eccentric, inspired, and provocative. He'd written eleven books by the time *The Body Has a Head* was published, including several plays and a biography of Noguchi, a Japanese playwright. Eckstein was more passionate about drama and literature than about human physiology, but his literary tour of the body brought that science to life for me.

I was an English major who until then had avoided science courses as if they carried lethal germs. Still, my father was a surgeon, and premeds swarmed the campus. I had taken a biology and a chemistry course "just in case" and didn't shine in either one. But Eckstein's book in one stroke overcame my naive fear of the culture of science and showed me a literary way to love the scientific side of medicine. And it planted that provocative title in my head. "The human mind is the body's master and the book's destination," Eckstein wrote in his introduction to *The Body Has a Head*.

My career has, in a roundabout way, chased that title, guided by the links between the mind and the body, between psychiatry and medicine, by the questions about how a mental illness affects a physical illness, and how to doctor them both. To me there is still no more fascinating territory in medicine, or in life, than the borderland between the mind and the body. The body has a head, and the heart has a brain. We know a lot about each, though less about the brain and how it runs things, like the heart, than about the rest of the body. Still, we know more about depression and heart disease than we do about the relationship of any other mental illness with any other physical illness, maybe because separately each illness is so common, so disabling, and sometimes deadly. The field of depression and heart disease happens to be the clinical territory where we're beginning to learn how a disorder of the mind translates into a disorder of the body, and the reverse. And one thing we keep learning over and over is how tricky it can be, in a life that is loaded with stresses—and whose isn't?—to spot either depression or heart disease early enough. Unless we're looking for them, they seem to sneak up on us like phantoms.

Murder in the Heart

"When my father fired me in 1990," Ted O'Reilly, fifty-six, remembers, "I was devastated. It hurt—hurt worse than anything I'd ever experienced. I was ready to . . . to commit murder." That was twelve years ago. He can smile about it now.

At fourteen, Teddy O'Reilly started drinking alone in his bedroom every night. "I could take a trip without ever leaving my bedroom," he says now. "I drank to escape."

Escape what?

"I don't know. Overbearing parents . . . dark feelings. Drinking made the dark feelings go away, for a while." His mother was drinking plenty herself at the time, several martinis on the porch every evening before joining his father for a few more and a late dinner. If they ever noticed Teddy sneaking their vodka and bourbon, they never mentioned it to him. Teddy hid bottles in his locker at school and drank between classes. His teachers commented sometimes on his odd behavior but never noticed his drinking. Quietly he drank through his teens and twenties, all the time doing well in school and eventually earning two masters degrees, the first in environmental engineering and the second in business administration.

During Teddy's teens and twenties his father had built a "fabulously successful" business career as an independent sales representative in the plastics industry. Teddy, the oldest of three, watched and waited. "It was tough as kids," Ted remembers. "He didn't have time for us. He had a terrible temper. In high school it was always strained with him. My friends were never good enough. When I married Sheila, she wasn't good enough for them. Hell, my parents wouldn't talk to us for three years after we got married. Three years." The ice broke only in his late twenties after his father had a serious accident and a long period of convalescence. Then he asked for help from Ted and his wife, who gave it. After his father recovered, Ted and Sheila left Indianapolis and headed west to Topeka. For Ted, it was an escape, but only a geographical one; he went to work for the company his father had represented for many years, hoping to earn the directorship of a regional office.

Topeka was good to Ted. He had ten happy years as a sales engineer, lots of friends, two kids, a fun-loving wife, good money, and time to hunt and fish. But when he saw that he was not destined to earn the directorship of a regional office, he looked around for options. His father, with whom he was speaking only a couple of times a year, had just retired and was looking for projects. When he invited Ted to start a business with him, Ted jumped at the offer. "I thought he was king," he said. With his father financing the start-up, they would manufacture and sell high-quality industrial plastic coatings. "He knew how to make it," Ted said of his father. "He would take me under his wing, but it would be my business. Didn't seem risky at all. The relationship actually worked okay for the first six months. It was when the business became successful that it started to change."

Within three years the company made reliable profits, but the tangle of family relationships tightened around Ted. "It was horrible," he said. "Dad demanded that my brother and sister be paid on the company payroll. Neither had ever done a damn thing, never worked at the company or anywhere else. Both had bad drug problems going back to their early twenties, and he was forcing me to subsidize them. The business was plenty successful, but he kept telling me how to do it better. Our profits were never good enough. I was never good enough. One day he asked me again what I was going to do to make the business grow, and I said, 'What would satisfy you?' He couldn't give me an answer. Silence. Same old stuff. Never good enough."

By the mid-1980s the business was doing well, but Ted was not. He remembers "the big dark cloud" dropping over him without warning. "Nothing made me happy. My secretary said to me one day, 'You just handed me the biggest order we've ever received and no smile?' I was getting no joy out of anything. My wife had to beg me to smile. I was tired most of the time, sleeping badly. Terrible." But he struggled on, assuming that because he could still work, he didn't need help with whatever this was. He wouldn't call it by name.

Clinical Tip 2.1: Know the warning signs of depression. Like many well-educated people, Ted missed signs of his depression for many years. If you don't know what to look for, you'll miss it. And you can't always count on your doctor, even some of the good ones, to raise the issue of watching out for warning signs of depression. The hallmark of major depression is two weeks or more of either feeling depressed, down, or hopeless most of the time, or feeling little interest or pleasure in doing things. In addition, look for trouble with sleep, appetite, concentration, memory, energy, and thoughts about death. Trouble in three or more of these areas for several weeks should raise a red flag and lead to an evaluation by a primary care doctor or a mental health specialist.[1]

Ted thought of himself as "stressed out." The concept of stress and its relationship to heart disease makes easy, intuitive sense. It pops up on the covers of *Time* and *Newsweek*. The American Heart Association tip sheets warn against stress. But the concept of stress sells better to the consumer than to the scientist. Stress is a scientifically slippery idea because we haven't measured it in a single standard fashion. Stress means too many things. We have used stress to mean both a stimulus and a response. We have used stress to mean a demanding event, like getting fired by your father or losing a child. And we have used stress to mean the anxious response to that demanding event, the syndrome of sweaty palms and racing heart and dry mouth and taut muscles. Under the umbrella of stress we think of the conditions that gnaw at our lives, such as poverty or a hostile marriage or night-shift work or big-city living in high-crime districts. And under this umbrella come the mental illnesses that make us anxious and "stressed out," like panic disorder, post-traumatic stress disorder, or major depression. All these stress-related events, responses, conditions, and illnesses dump excessive demands on our stress-response system, the system that usually orchestrates our body's resilient response to challenges. The cumulative burden of these challenges to our stress-response system is called the allostatic load, and this new concept is the focus of some of the most promising stress research.[2] When this system gets overwhelmed, we get sick, mentally and often physically.

Understanding the size of the problem of stress and heart disease begins with defining at least a part of this large and ungainly puzzle, and then attempting to measure it in some epidemiologic fashion. If we think of clinical depression as a final common pathway for many stress-related problems—and one that we can measure and do something about—then focusing on depression provides a way to begin estimating how many people are affected by clinically meaningful persistent distress and heart disease. So how do we find these people?

The Low Point

In 1988 Ted decided to stop drinking, hoping that would make the difference. He went to AA, quit drinking, and for five years attended four or five AA meetings a week. He was surprised by how easy it was to quit drinking, "easier than quitting smoking." Ted had smoked since his early teens, first cigarettes and then cigars, every day. He still smokes cigars ("I like the cheap ones, King Edwards. Sheila thinks I inhale, but I don't, not much.") After he quit drinking, instead of improving, he felt worse—anxious, unhappy, angry—and was sleeping badly, so he sought the help of a psychologist once a week for six months and started a low dose of imipramine, an antidepressant medication. Then in 1990 his father fired him.

"That was the worst, the lowest point in my life," Ted said. "For weeks I wanted to kill that man. . . . I staked out my parents' office. I had a plan for getting a gun. I was that bad off. Nothing else mattered. The only thing that saved me from doing it was that they moved to Arizona. That saved me. I was relieved. I'd never, never wanted to kill anybody. That wasn't me. And never since, but right then I could have."

Ted's psychologist told him he was depressed and put him in the hospital. The two-week hospitalization didn't have much effect. The doctor made a minor change in his medication but told him his depression was "environmental" and he'd have to try to change his circumstances. He left the hospital feeling almost as depressed as when he went in. He didn't stay on the medicine more than a few weeks, but after about three months he began to immerse himself in starting a new business that would compete directly with his father's plastics operation. He launched this company within a year of losing his job, and three months later he turned a profit. Was he afire with revenge? Or with entrepreneurial talent that could not be crushed? His company has earned profits each of the last eleven years, netting him more than a million dollars a year for the last six.

But this success didn't solve his problems and it didn't lift the depression. Ted continued to be dogged by fatigue. He took no pleasure in the growth of his business or in his family's social life. And he ceased to care whether he lived or died. In 1993 at the age of forty-six, Ted O'Reilly was simply going though the motions. And now, on top of his general fatigue, he began having fleeting waves of total exhaustion, just for a few minutes, collapsing him in his tracks. What was that?

Facing Risks

Over the last forty years epidemiologic studies have taught us a lot about the risks for heart disease, and this science of risk management has seeped into the American culture.[3] We now know, for example, that, six mutable risk factors (factors about which we can do something) exert a major effect on our chances of developing the most common form of heart disease, coronary disease: abnormal lipids, high blood pressure, smoking, diabetes, physical inactivity, and obesity.[4] Each of these factors independently adds to our risk, and reducing or eliminating any one of them reduces our risk for either developing coronary disease or dying from it. We now have butt huts and bans on smoking indoors, exercise rooms in office buildings, and ads for cholesterol-lowering drugs on the evening news.

As obvious and conventional as this may seem to us now, thirty years ago we didn't know with scientific conviction that lowering blood pressure to normal would reduce our risk of death by 20 percent or that quitting smoking could reduce our risk of coronary disease by half within a year.[5]

Major Risk Factors for Coronary Disease

Fixed Risks
   Older age (over 40)
   Male sex
   Family history of heart disease
Changeable Risks
   Smoking
   High blood pressure
   Abnormal lipids
      Elevated LDL cholesterol
      Decreased HDL cholesterol
      Elevated triglycerides
   Diabetes
   Obesity
   Physical inactivity

Clinical Tip 2.2: Know your risks for heart disease.

Men in their forties and women in their fifties are approaching the age when coronary disease develops. If you don't know how you're doing on the six major risk factors, you don't have much chance of preventing heart disease. Most of us would prefer not to think about it until we have to—I waited until I was fifty-two to get my worrisome numbers—but if we wait until symptoms force us to face the problem, much of the damage will already have been done. How's your blood pressure? What's your LDL cholesterol? How much exercise do you get each week? Is that enough? What's your BMI (body mass index)? What's your fasting blood sugar? How old were your relatives when they got heart disease? Most of us don't bother asking these questions until it's too late. But timely answers could save your life or save you lots of grief, if you're willing to change your ways to reduce your cardiac risk. Check the American Heart Association's website to start sizing up your risk (*www.americanheart.org*, search Risk Assessment), and talk to your doctor.

And twenty years ago we thought all cholesterol was bad; now we know that one type of cholesterol (low-density lipoprotein, or LDL) raises risk and another type (high density lipoprotein, or HDL) lowers risk.

Knowledge is power, and the power of this epidemiologic knowledge about heart disease has driven the dramatic drop in the death rate for coronary disease in the United States since around 1980. But we also know that these risk factors explain less than half the new cases of coronary disease. Our predictions have improved a lot over half a century, but heart disease is still something of a crapshoot. Plenty of people with multiple risk factors never have heart attacks, and plenty of people with heart attacks have few or no traditional risk factors. About half of all men and over 60 percent of all women who die from heart attacks had no symptoms of heart disease before the attack.[6] Does adding depression to the prediction process improve our understanding of heart disease?

Clinical Tip 2.3: Know the warning signs of heart disease.
And remember that depression may make it harder to recognize them. For men, the common signs are chest pains with exertion, easy fatigability, and shortness of breath. For women, the common signs are more likely to feel like indigestion, as well as sudden fatigue and trouble breathing. Depression confuses the picture by causing fatigue and chest pain and indigestion.

Consider Ted O'Reilly in 1993 at forty-six. Was he worrying about heart disease? No, he was worrying about whether he could get out of bed each morning, about how to fake a smile, about where the juice and joy of life had gone. Neither his doctor nor his wife, Sheila, was worrying about his heart either. Ted didn't fit the profile. He had none of the common symptoms of heart disease, such as chest pain with exercise or shortness of breath. Aside from smoking a few cigars a day, what risk factors did he have? None that he knew about. He hadn't bothered to check his cholesterol. He'd never had a chronic illness. He took no medications. His mind was on his business and his misery.

One day in 1993 while Ted was walking across the plant, a walk he had made daily in the year since the plant opened, he suddenly felt so exhausted he had to stop and sit down. Then the feeling passed. Two months later, again without warning or apparent cause, exhaustion overtook him for a few fleeting moments as he carried some luggage in an airport. He had to sit down. Almost missed his plane. No chest pains, no lasting effects, just the fleeting wave of exhaustion.

In March 1994, while Ted fiddled in his garden one afternoon, doing nothing strenuous:

> I got this terrible feeling, pain in both shoulders and in my neck and my jaw. I thought, 'This is weird, or this is a heart attack.' I went inside and tried to take a shower and relax, but it wouldn't go away, so I told my son I was driving myself to the hospital. When they saw my EKG, that emergency room started hopping and I was terrified. I asked a chaplain standing in the hall if he was there because of me and he said no, but I was terrified. They gave me TPA [an enzyme that dissolves clots] and I spent a night in the ICU and the next day my angiogram only showed 60 percent blockage in one vessel, so the cardiologist told me I probably had spasm in that vessel and he could treat me just with drugs. My cholesterol was way up there too, 260, I think, so I started on Lipitor to bring it down, and aspirin. And I started exercising. He told me to quit smoking, but I didn't.

Here, Ted smiled like a child shrugging off his parent.

> I did fine for about eight months until I got these scary sharp neck pains, always on my left, shooting up at my head, always when I was doing something physical, especially jogging. So my cardiologist got me on the treadmill test and they pushed me and I didn't feel good at the time, but they said everything looked fine, so what could I do? I walked away and then, before I could get to my car, I started to feel worse, a lot worse—pain, that exhaustion again, just bad. I turned around and walked back in there and they put the EKG on me and everyone started jumping into action when they saw my strip. I was terrified, worse this time, shaking all over. My legs were so out of control they had to pin me down. They gave me TPA again and put me in the hospital and the next day they did an angioplasty to open that artery up. I've been fine ever since. That was eight years ago.

Ted's second angiogram reported narrowing at two sites along the same artery that had given him the heart attack earlier that year. When his heart first troubled him, high levels of cholesterol had likely been flowing in his blood for many years and his smoking had been aggravating his cardiovascular system since his early teens. He'd worked a sedentary job for years and had no hobbies that demanded exertion, having given up hunting and fishing. But he was free of diabetes, hypertension, and obesity. Heart disease had spared his parents and close relatives. What stands out most in his medical history prior to his heart attack in 1993 is his long history of alcohol dependence and about ten years of struggling with depression, a struggle that heated up when he stopped drinking. Though it's not yet possible to quantify depression's contribution to cardiac risk, it's likely that Ted O'Reilly's depression added to the risk he had already incurred by his smoking, high cholesterol, and physical inactivity.

Treatment That Works

In addition to identifying cardiac risks, we've learned a lot over the past several decades about the risks for depression, and this aspect of psychiatric epidemiology has also changed our culture. We now know that all over the world women suffer from depression more often than men. Genes play a substantial role in the risk for depression, and a greater role in severe than in mild depression. So a family history of depression may be a risk factor. And age counts too. In the United States over the past fifty years, rates of depression have risen dramatically. A person born between 1966 and 1975 now has three to four times the risk for a depressive episode of a person born between 1946 and 1956, five times the risk of a person born between 1936 and 1945. Smoking is associated with high rates of depression. So are diabetes, chronic pain, and most chronic physical illnesses.[7] So age, gender, family history, substance abuse, and chronic illness are all risk factors for depression.

Fifteen years ago we knew none of this about the risks for clinical depression. Now we have National Depression Screening Day every October, and in November politicians win elections in spite of admitting to taking Prozac. Celebrities tell us about their struggles with depression and other mental illnesses. Everybody knows what Prozac is, and three of the ten most often prescribed medications in the United States are antidepressants. This is the power of scientific knowledge translated into action on a national scale to change culture and, we hope, to improve health.

It took Ted O'Reilly fourteen years to find effective treatment for his depression. Once he found it, he knew within a month that the treatment was working. In 1997 his cardiologist referred him to Dr Barbara Ritchken, a psychiatrist on the other side of town. She's a middle-aged woman who speaks a South African brand of the Queen's English and conducts her therapy sessions with a no-nonsense blend of pragmatic advice, empathic psychotherapy, and energetic medication management. She told Ted on his first visit that he had severe and chronic depression and had had it for many years, possibly since before he started drinking as a teenager.[8] She prescribed twenty milligrams of paroxetine (Paxil), the starting dose of a common antidepressant, and the two began meeting weekly for individual cognitive therapy focused on managing Ted's depression. The symptoms lifted within a month and he's had no depressive episodes since. After a year he reduced his therapy sessions to several times a year, and he still takes the same dose of Paxil.

Clinical Tip 2.4: Insist on effective treatment for depression.
Depression makes it tough to recover from heart disease. If you have heart disease and symptoms of depression, insist on effective treatment of your depression. Your aim as a measure of full recovery should be no depressive symptoms for at least two months. For too long, Ted O'Reilly did not know what adequate or effective treatment of depression meant for him or how to get it. Once he recovered from his depression eight years after he first sought treatment, his heart disease became relatively easy to manage. Though it's not always possible to eliminate all symptoms of depression, you and your doctor should know what the standards for adequate treatment of depression are and how to get more intensive treatment if your first efforts don't result in a full recovery from depression.[9]

When I asked what he believed about why he had his first heart attack in 1993, Ted O'Reilly said, without hesitating, "The stress of losing my job in 1990, serious stress." For him it's a reasonable guess that "serious stress," his catch-all phrase for his relationship with his father, his firing, and his depression, combined with high cholesterol and smoking to shut down his coronary artery through a combination of atherosclerosis and spasm in the artery.

His total cholesterol this year was 147, down to normal from the high 200s. Several exercise stress tests for his heart over the past several years have been normal. And his annual cardiac evaluations tell him he's doing well. For now, at fifty-six, he has beaten the triple afflictions of alcoholism, depression, and coronary disease. Over the past five years Ted has been free of symptoms and has been "loving life." Several years ago he and Sheila bought a house in the Ozarks, where he's back to trout fishing. Others run the daily operations of his business for him. And he still defiantly enjoys a few King Edward cigars every day.

Counting the Odds

How many people like Ted O'Reilly (and like Tom Geraci and Paula Volk in Chapter 1) are affected by both depression and heart disease? What has our knowledge of the epidemiology of heart disease and the epidemiology of depression taught us about who might develop both depression and heart disease? The answers to these questions would be straightforward if epidemiologic studies of heart disease had also looked carefully at depression, or if epidemiologic studies of depression had also looked at heart disease, but so far that hasn't happened at a level of scientific rigor that would answer the questions directly and reliably. But these two fields of investigation have begun to overlap, and from recent studies we can estimate how many people are likely to be affected by depression and heart disease and who's at risk.

First, a word of caution when talking about risks. Epidemiology is the science of how illness affects large numbers of people. Epidemiology's interest in large numbers means it deals in probabilities, and it manages uncertainties. It's a science of conjecture, a discipline of educated guesses about probabilities of health and illness. Jimmy the Greek at the bedside. Approximations, estimates, ranges, odds—these comprise the street talk for discussing risks for illness. Such terms imply guesswork and the possibility of error, but they are the honest way to talk about trends in complex illnesses over large populations where certainty can't be had.

From the National Comobidity Survey, generally considered the best study of mental illness in a representative sample of the general population of the United States, we know that one in four of the U.S. citizens surveyed reported some form of depressive disorder in their lifetimes. During any given year about fourteen million adults experience the more severe form, major depression. That makes severe depression one of the most common major illnesses in the United States, as common as the most common form of heart disease, coronary disease.[10]

The American Heart Association estimates that the number of U.S. citizens affected in a given year by all types of cardiovascular disease is about 71 million, more than a quarter of the adult population. Of these 71 million, many have high blood pressure only, but about 16 million have one of the two most common forms of heart disease—coronary disease or congestive heart failure.[11]

By any measure of public health, depression and heart disease stand out among the most common illnesses, both in the United States and worldwide. Depression and heart disease each afflict about 25 percent of the U.S. adult population at some time in their lives.

We know from studies of clinical populations—that is, people who seek treatment—that depression is about three times more common in people who seek treatment for heart disease than in the general population.

Table 2.1. Frequency of Selected Cardiovascular Diseases in the United States, 2006

Condition	%	Prevalence
High blood pressure	31.0	65,000,000
Coronary heart disease	6.3	13,200,000
Stroke	2.6	5,500,000
Heart failure	2.4	5,000,000
Congenital heart defects	0.5	1,000,000
All cardiovascular diseases	34.2	71,300,000*

Source: Adapted from Thom (2006). See also Labarthe, *Epidemiology and Prevention of Cardiovascular Diseases.*

*Based on the estimated number of persons affected, taking into account the occurrence of multiple conditions in the same person.

The frequency of current major depression ranges from 16–22 percent in patients hospitalized after a heart attack, compared to 5–8 percent in the general population. The rate of major depression in patients with congestive heart failure is also about 20 percent. We can guess from these clinical studies that of the 16 million adults in the United States who have coronary disease or congestive heart failure during a year, at least 16 percent, or 2.6 million, have current major depression. That's more than twice the number of people who have strokes in a given year.

Alexander Glassman, MD, has another way of estimating the size of the problem. As a professor of psychiatry at Columbia University and the lead author on the largest and most rigorous study of an antidepressant medication for depression after a heart attack, Dr. Glassman says: "Consider that every year about 1.5 million people in the United States have either a heart attack or an episode of chest pain related to heart disease that forces them into the hospital. About 40 percent or 600,000 of them will have severe or moderate depression within a month of this episode, and that depression will triple their risk of dying within six months." That's the size of the most urgent part of the problem of depression and heart disease in the United States—more than half a million people each year.[12]

Two other depression groups contribute to the size of the problem, though their numbers are less clear because they have not been as well studied in groups with heart disease: people who have had an episode of major depression in the past, and people with minor depression now or in the past. As we'll see in the next chapter, focusing only on those who currently have major depression ignores two facts: depressions come and go, and for most people depression is a recurrent illness with long intervals between episodes. Asking only about current depression, as most studies have done, taps about a third of those with recurrent depression and ignores the majority, those affected over long periods. There is also evidence that minor depression, which affects about 10 percent of the general population and 20 percent of the heart disease population, raises the early mortality rates of heart disease. Studies that ignore minor depression underestimate the true effect of depression on heart disease.

Arguing for a broader concept than clinical depression alone, a psychologist from the Netherlands, Johan Denollet, has proposed the type D personality, a set of traits that combine a pattern of anxious and depressive feelings with a tendency toward social inhibition and isolation. Denollet has shown that people who score high on the fourteen-item type D questionnaire have higher rates of death from coronary disease than those who score low. He argues that what damages the cardiovascular system is not just depression or feeling bad, but feeling bad alone over many years, that is, without the buffer of easy expression and friends to take the edge off.[13]

So, when we ask how big a public health problem the combination of stress, depression, and heart disease is, the answer depends on how broadly we define stress or depression, where we set the threshold of concern, and how much we consider the duration and the severity of the clinical depression. The answer also depends on what we define as heart disease. Our discussion so far has ignored stroke and hypertension and arrhythmias and rheumatic heart disease when they occur separately from coronary disease or congestive heart failure, because they are diseases for which we have too few good data on the rates of coexisting depression.

The narrower estimate, for which we have sound science, focuses on the 600,000 people each year with clinical depression soon after a heart attack or severe chest pain as the group deserving the most urgent concern because of their high early death rates. On the other hand, the broadest estimate of depressive disorders over a lifetime, including major and minor depression, current and past, suggests that depression could affect 40 percent of the population that has coronary disease or congestive heart failure—at least seven million people. To understand the true size of this public health problem, we need to study these other categories of chronic stress, depression, and heart disease more carefully. In the meantime, who are these seven million people who may be affected? And more urgently, who are the 600,000 who have a heightened risk of dying in the coming year?

CHAPTER 3

Converging Risks

To understand who gets caught in the crossfire of depression and heart disease, two seemingly separate illnesses—one mental and the other physical, one striking young and the other striking old, one episodic and the other chronic, one in the brain and the other in the heart—we have to understand the risks for each condition. Then it becomes clear how the risks for depression converge on the risks for heart disease, setting up the cycle that hastens the progression of each condition.

Depression

The age at which most people first develop depression, the midtwenties, is about three decades younger than the age at which most people develop the common forms of heart disease. And this age of onset for depression has been dropping rapidly in the United States, as well as around the world. The National Comorbidity Survey (NCS), its first wave completed in 1992, the best continuing study of mental illness in the general population of the United States, looked at the change in rates of depression over a period of forty years. Figure 3.1 reflects some of the findings: People born between 1936 and 1945 in the United States had roughly a 5 percent chance of having had a depressive episode by age twenty, compared to a 35 percent chance for the group born between 1966 and 1975.[1] That's a steep and steady climb.

Sadly, we don't know why the rates of depression have risen so dramatically. Better diagnostic methods explain only a small portion of the rise. Some experts cite a parallel rise in substance abuse rates. Others note the rise in divorce rates and in the mobility of the American family,

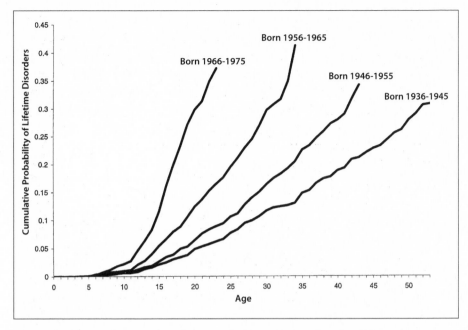

Figure 3.1. Age of Onset for Major and Minor Depression by Cohort in the 1992 National Comorbidity Survey. Rates of depression rose steadily during the last half of the twentieth century.

which contribute to losses and decreased social support, a pattern of social fragmentation.

This recent rise in the rates of depression means that more and more of the people now approaching the age of greatest risk for developing heart disease, their fifties and sixties, will have had depression for longer periods of their lives prior to developing heart disease. If depression had an important effect on heart disease ten and twenty years ago, it is more important now because of the larger numbers affected for longer periods.

Women run a greater risk for depression than men in every country and culture studied. In one review, the female-to-male ratio for major depression varied from 1.6:1 in Taiwan and Lebanon to 3.1:1 in West Germany. That means that at least one and a half times as many women as men had serious depression in Taiwan, but in Germany it was three times as many women as men. In the United States the ratio was 2.6:1 based on data collected around 1980, and 1.7:1 based on data collected around 2002.[2] This cruel favoring of women shows up as early as age ten and persists until age fifty, that is, in women of child-bearing age. After that the ratio returns to 1:1.

Why women of childbearing age? Women don't fare worse than men with respect to how chronic their depression is or their speed of recovery or their response to treatment. That is, once depression strikes, women do about as well—or as poorly—as men. Most of the higher risk for women results from their higher risk for the first few episodes in their younger years.

No one has established the basis for this gender difference in depression. There are many proposed explanations, but the leading contributing factors include: (a) shifts in sex hormones during puberty, menstrual periods, pregnancy, and menopause; (b) genes; and (c) social factors, such as the demands of mothering and physical or sexual abuse. The importance of this gender difference in depression for the later development of heart dis-

Table 3.1. Female/Male Ratio of Major Depression in Ten Countries

	Female/Male Ratio	Rate of Major Depression (%)
Germany	3.1	9.2
Italy	3.0	12.4
USA	2.6	5.2
France	2.1	16.4
New Zealand	2.1	11.6
Korea	2.0	2.9
Canada	1.9	9.6
Puerto Rico	1.8	4.3
Lebanon	1.6	19.0
Taiwan	1.6	1.5

Source: Weissman, Bland, Canino, et al., 1996.
Note: The rates of depression in the table are those of the country's general population, ages eighteen to sixty-four.

ease comes with the greater exposure to depression of some women before they develop signs of heart disease. If exposure to depression increases the chances of developing heart disease, then this effect should be greater for women than for men and greatest in women with long or severe histories of depression.[3]

Relatives of people with severe or chronic depression are at risk. In the United States, if you've never had depression but you have a first-degree relative (parent, sibling, or child) with a depressive disorder, your chances of developing a depressive disorder are about three times greater than if none of your first-degree relatives had depression. The family of the great novelist Henry James had a genetic vulnerability to severe depression that showed up in his father, himself, and three of his four siblings, sparing only his mother and one brother. I've treated patients who can trace depression through three and sometimes four generations of their families. This familial risk remains even if you were adopted and raised away from your biological parents, so most of this risk is genetic. We don't yet know which genes do the damage, but because depression, like heart disease, is the result of a complex set of factors and consists of several types, its hereditary risk is unlikely ever to be reduced to a single gene. Large and rigorous studies to search for specific sets of genes for depression began only in 2000 and have not yet clarified the genetic risk. Whether the genes for depression bear any relationship to the genes for heart disease remains to be discovered.[4]

Depression leads to depression. Previous episodes of depression raise our risk for a future episode. Half of all people who have one episode of major depression will suffer a second episode sometime in their lives, and of those who have a second, 75 percent will have a third. After three episodes the likelihood of further episodes jumps to 90 percent without preventive treatment.[5] Depression seems to get worse with practice; or, the longer it goes on, the harder it may become to control it. This pattern of persistent or recurrent depression is more likely to hasten or worsen heart disease than one or two brief episodes.

Stressful events trigger some episodes of depression, but mostly in the early stages of depressive disorders. That is, your first depressive episode is more likely to be precipitated by stressful events than is your tenth episode.[6] I took care of a first-year college student who came to me late in September, suicidal after getting a C in her first chemistry exam. This

"A-student" had had a previous milder depression, and her response to her exam grade triggered her first major depressive episode. This stronger effect of adverse events early in the course of a recurrent depressive illness may reflect the fact that, once established, recurrent depression can take on a life of its own, and the timing of episodes then depends less on external events than on internal factors, such as the way one thinks or sleeps or manages conflict at work. As with Paula Volk in Chapter 1, a heart attack or a coronary bypass operation may serve as a stressful and precipitating event for a first depressive episode.

Even more than single stressful events, chronic anxiety disorders, such as panic disorder, add to the risk for depression. And people who have both depression and panic disorder, a fairly common combination, have a higher risk of developing heart disease than people who have only depression or only panic disorder.[7]

Chronic medical illnesses deliver plenty of stressful events in the form of bad news, pain, surgery, loss of work, and sometimes loss of friends. In general, chronic illnesses roughly double the risk for depression. People with heart disease, diabetes, or high blood pressure consistently report higher rates of depression than do people with no chronic illness. And that effect remains true independent of the effects of other factors which might account for the higher depression rates, such as age, smoking, poverty, or physical inactivity, all of which are also associated with both chronic illness and depression. In fact, the effect of chronic medical illness extends beyond depression, raising the risk for common mental illnesses in general, including anxiety disorders and substance abuse.[8]

The way medical illnesses, such as heart disease, contribute to mental illnesses still eludes simple explanations. The mechanisms are likely to be complex and to vary from illness to illness, but all chronic illnesses impose persistent, often daily demands on the central nervous system to manage, for example, an overworked heart or a depleted pancreas or a low pain threshold in the spine. That wear and tear eventually may expose the inherent genetic vulnerabilities of the brain and mind to develop a mental illness. Depression is one way the brain tires out. In addition, often these chronic medical illnesses cut people off from friends or rob them of their jobs and self-esteem. When these medical illnesses interfere with sleep and sex and fun, they pave the way for depression. And some depressions induced by a

Risk Factors for Major Depression

Female sex
Family history of depression
Previous episodes of major depression
Severe stressful events
Persistent stressful conditions
>Poverty
>Physical or sexual abuse
>Other chronic psychiatric illnesses
>Anxiety
>Substance abuse
>Chronic medical illness

Clinical Tip 3.1: Know your risks for depression. The list above summarizes the risk factors for major depression. What is your family history of depression? How many previous episodes of depression have you had—treated or untreated? Consider the significance of your age and gender when you assess the impact of stressful events, physical illness, substance abuse, and smoking on your risk for depression. Talk to your doctor or mental health specialist to understand whether you have a low, medium, or high risk for depression.

---

medical illness can be effectively treated by treating the underlying medical illness.

So depression favors the young and women and family members of the depressed. Within a lifetime, one spell of depression raises the chances of another, and stressful events often catalyze the process through the first episode or two, after which it takes on a life of its own and needs less and less catalyzing. Poverty, substance abuse, and physical illnesses like heart disease all hammer away at the central nervous system, exposing genetic and learned tendencies toward depression.

Heart Disease

The early signs of the common heart diseases—coronary disease and congestive heart failure—usually begin in the fifties for men and sixties for women, three to four decades later than the early signs of depression. After age fifty, the risk for heart disease rises with age. But for most heart diseases the pathologic processes begin years, sometimes decades, before any signs or symptoms declare the illness. Ted O'Reilly's heart attack was only the sudden outcome of many years of slow and silent corrosion in his artery walls. But this process is visible only to researchers; it remains invisible to the patient and the doctor. New vascular-imaging scans can now identify the early stages of the disease process of atherosclerosis or the laying down of hard plaques in the arteries as early as the twenties and thirties. Without high-tech imaging, it's hard for clinicians to find evidence of the early stages of heart disease before age forty.

Compared to the linear increase in risk with age, the effect of gender on cardiac risk is trickier. Coronary disease affects as many women as men, but men develop coronary disease about a decade younger and die from it younger than women. Instead of the well-known crushing chest pain so typical in men, symptoms of a heart attack in women tend to feature palpitations, dizziness, nausea, and fatigue, symptoms that can often be mistaken for anxiety. Because in women the narrowing of the arteries often occurs in smaller arteries of the heart than in men, traditional angiograms may miss coronary disease more frequently in women.

On the other hand, once women in the United States get coronary disease, they tend to die sooner in the hospital after heart attacks, angioplasty, and bypass surgery than men do. These higher death rates for women may be related to the fact that, for a variety of social reasons, women in the United States have traditionally received less aggressive treatment for heart disease than men have. Women are less likely than men are to get cardiac rehabilitation, coronary bypass surgery, and heart transplants. Until menopause, their hormones protect women somewhat from coronary disease, but after menopause their rates rise to match men's. And any protective effect from hormones in women before menopause vanishes with either smoking or diabetes.[9]

In spite of the distinct differences in gender effects on coronary disease and on depression, no consistent pattern of gender effects has emerged in studies of combined depression and coronary disease. The inconsistencies may reflect the complex effects of depression on the traditional cardiac risk factors that vary with gender. For example, smoking is a greater cardiac risk factor for men, whereas diabetes is a greater risk factor for women.[10] As in the general population, depression is more common in women with heart disease than in men with heart disease. And in the United States, while mortality rates from heart disease have steadily declined for men over the past twenty years, mortality rates for women have risen slightly.[11]

Like depression, heart disease runs in families. Patterns of extremes (either lots of relatives with heart disease, or none) help predict risk. And age of onset in the family history is important too, since people who get heart disease at forty-five carry greater risks for their relatives than do those who get it at ninety. Genes clearly play a strong role, but, as with depression, our environment heavily influences whether we develop the heart disease for which we may be genetically vulnerable.

So age, gender, and family history are the three most important cardiac risk factors that we can't do anything about. The six major risk factors for coronary disease that we can change, listed in Chapter 2, are substantially influenced by depression. Through these influences the risks for depression converge on the risks for heart disease. The strongest link is with smoking.

Clinical Tip 3.2: Learn how depression affects your risks for heart disease. Use the following sections to discuss with your doctor whether depression is raising any of your risks for heart disease. If so, find out how treating the depression may make it easier to manage your heart disease risks.

Depression and Smoking

Smoking is bad for heart disease, but for people with a history of depression smoking is even worse. A study of 1,100 men in the San Francisco area found that depression tripled the effect of smoking on the degree of atherosclerosis. If smoking is bad for plaque formation, smoking plus depression is three times as bad. (In this study, depression also magnified the effect of cholesterol on atherosclerosis.)[12]

Depression drives some people to start smoking, and depression makes it much tougher for smokers to quit. Studies have consistently shown that smokers report higher rates of depression than nonsmokers. For many veteran smokers who attempt to quit, depression lurks like the wolf at the door. Smoking keeps depression at bay. I talked to a man recently who at forty-nine has had two heart attacks followed by congestive heart failure and depression. He figures his heart is so weak that he has only "another five to seven years to live." He told me he's done everything his doctors suggested to improve his heart disease (lowered his cholesterol, attended cardiac rehabilitation programs, diligently taken his cardiac medications), but he has not been able to quit smoking. He's tried to quit many times, by will power and with the help of medications and a nicotine patch, but he turns so nasty and irritable and anxious and depressed when he quits that he can't go on. And nothing relieves this torture as fast and as effectively as a cigarette. He regrets the smoking, but he fears more the effect of quitting. His wife and kids hate watching him smoke. It looks like slow suicide. He feels trapped.

Some intriguing biology may explain this pernicious pairing of curses. Nicotine facilitates the release of three neurotransmitters that play major roles in recovery from depression—dopamine, serotonin, and norepinephrine—as we will see in Chapter 4. Nicotine also affects the cholinergic system in parts of the brain that play key roles in depression (the hippocampus, the locus coeruleus, and the amygdala, for instance). And nicotine increases the expression of brain-derived neurotrophic factor (BDNF), a substance that plays a key role in recovery from depression. By these pathways, for many smokers with a history of depression, nicotine functions as a short-acting antidepressant, much the way other stimulants such as Dexedrine, caffeine, and cocaine can.[13]

While nicotine may protect some people against depression, smoking fuels the smoldering fire of heart disease by (a) hastening the hardening of the arteries through atherosclerosis, (b) causing spasm in the coronary arteries, (c) promoting small clots to form, (d) disrupting the rhythms of the heart, and (e) making it harder for the red blood cells to carry oxygen.[14] Smoking is a dangerous trade-off, rushing frequent boosts to the brain at some later cost to the heart. For people who have experienced depression, smoking offers protection from the more urgent threat of unbearable withdrawal and a return to depression. So depression indirectly contributes to heart disease by making it doubly tough for smokers with a history of depression to quit.

Depression and Diabetes

Depression is common in diabetes. About one in four people with diabetes have moderate to severe depressive symptoms, and one in ten have a full depressive disorder. As with other chronic illnesses, people with diabetes have about twice the chance of being depressed as people without diabetes. Diabetes is hard enough to manage when you're up, but it's harder to manage when you're down. For a variety of reasons, depression makes it harder to control blood sugar, and depression is associated with diabetic complications such as kidney disease, vision loss, and peripheral nerve damage. Once it occurs in the context of diabetes, depression lasts longer and recurs more frequently than depression in people without diabetes.[15]

So depression is bad for diabetes and diabetes is bad for heart disease, and diabetes is especially bad for heart disease in women. Compared to men with diabetes, women with diabetes tend to have more severe and diffuse atherosclerosis and higher rates of dying early after heart attacks. Depression may offer an explanation for why women with diabetes have such a hard time with coronary disease. Investigators at Washington University in St. Louis followed for ten years a group of adults with diabetes but initially no heart disease. The people with diabetes who also had depression histories were three times more likely to develop coronary disease than those who had never had depression. And for the women with diabetes, depression raised the risk of developing coronary disease by five times, compared to women with no depression. Even heavy smoking doesn't exacerbate cardiac risks that much. So depression magnifies the effect of diabetes on heart disease risk.[16]

Depression and Physical Inactivity

By any definition of physical inactivity (such as a sedentary job or no light exercise in the past week or no exertion greater than three kilocalories per minute in the last month), it nearly doubles the risk for coronary disease.[17] Idleness is toxic to arteries. Atherosclerosis dines on couch potatoes. And depression is the enemy of any activity, mental or physical.

Depressed people exercise less, feel less physical vigor, tire more easily, and have worse physical health than do people who are free of depression. The fatigue of depression shackles the most determined of its victims and often dominates the appearance of the depressed person. Picture the sagging shoulders, the listless gait, the droop of the eyelids and the corners of the mouth. The physical inactivity of depression reflects the mental shutdown.

On the other hand, many people with mild to moderate depression find that regular exercise, as little as half an hour of jogging three times a week, relieves depressive symptoms and may be as effective as medications or psychotherapy.[18] And sustained regular exercise is also good for heart disease, both its onset and its progression, although there's still debate about whether exercise reduces mortality. One of the cornerstones of cognitive therapy for depression focuses on increasing activity of all kinds, based on the observation that a depressed mood worsens with inactivity and improves with activity, especially pleasurable activity, whether mental or physical. What's good for the mind is good for the heart. So chronic or recurrent depression indirectly contributes to heart disease by reducing physical activity levels, often for months or years, sometimes playing a pivotal role in the drift toward a sedentary lifestyle.

Depression and Obesity

Does depression make people fat? It depends. Though many people lose their appetites and sometimes lose weight when depressed, some people eat more when they feel down. About a third of people seeking treatment for obesity in the United States report binge eating in association with high rates of depression. A well-described syndrome, atypical depression, is marked by overpowering cravings for sweets that often trigger eating binges, usually at night. It's not uncommon for people with atypical depressions to consume half gallons of ice cream or whole bags of candy in an hour.

The link between depression and obesity may begin early in life for children with major depression. A recent study at Columbia University followed a group of ninety children diagnosed with major depression, comparing them to a similar group of children who had no psychiatric illness. As young adults ten to fifteen years later, the group that had major depression in childhood had become significantly more overweight or obese. Both childhood depression and poverty predicted being overweight as an adult in this study, and the longer the depression lasted, the greater the chances of being overweight.[19]

Depression is rarely good for obesity. Dieting is tough work, and the behavior change required by any substantial weight-loss program calls for cognitive, emotional, and social discipline. Depression makes these changes tougher to initiate and tougher to hold on to, undermining the best efforts at dieting and other weight-loss regimens.[20]

So depression may contribute to heart disease by exacerbating obesity, particularly in people who develop depression in childhood and for whom depression leads to binge eating. One of the steps along the pathway from depression to heart disease is the recently described metabolic syndrome, a stress-related condition that includes a combination of diabetes, obesity, high blood pressure, and high lipids. (We'll see more about this in Chapter 7.)

Though some intriguing studies have begun to look at the link between depression and abnormal lipids and between depression and high blood pressure, depression does not directly exacerbate either of these risk factors. There is some evidence that depression predicts the later development of high blood pressure, but, on the whole, the research has been neither ample in volume nor conclusive in findings.[21]

Clinical Tip 3.3: Don't give up on changing risky behaviors.
Changing cardiac risk behaviors like smoking, overeating, and avoiding exercise can be tough and frustrating. Depression can make the task appear impossible. The most effective method for changing health behaviors is described in *Changing for Good*, by James Prochaska (1994). This readable self-help book can guide you and your doctor to develop a plan and help you stick to it until it works. If your doctor is not familiar with this method, ask for a referral to a social worker, psychologist, or psychiatrist who will work with you on changing these behaviors. Don't give up.

What does all this add up to? Depression is associated with at least four of the six major risk factors for coronary disease. Just by exacerbating the effects of these risk factors, depression may increase a person's vulnerability to coronary disease. Depression exacerbated Ted O'Reilly's smoking and reduced his physical activity. Aside from any direct influence depression might have on the course of coronary disease (more on that in Chapter 5), depression plays this pernicious and, until recently, unnoticed backstage role. It frustrates the smokers who try to quit, complicates the already complicated life of the diabetic, idles the sluggish, and adds pounds to the overweight. Depression throws fat into the fire of atherosclerosis.

So the people most at risk for developing both depression and heart disease are likely to be women, people who have had episodes of depression in the past, and people who have several current major cardiac risk factors. Often their families have suffered from depression or heart disease or both. In these ways the risks for depression, most of which have declared themselves in people's twenties and thirties, converge upon the risks for heart disease as they emerge into their forties and fifties. Persistent depression plays a setup role for heart disease.

Do these indirect effects fully explain depression's effect on heart disease? No. To understand the full effect of depression on heart disease, we have to understand what depression is and how it works in the mind, brain, and body.

CHAPTER 4

Depression: Disease
of Mind, Brain, and Body

If there be Hell upon earth, it's to be found
in a melancholy man's heart.
　　　—Robert Burton, *Anatomy of Melancholy*, 1621

Although in Robert Burton's day grave-digging amateur anatomists did try to find things like the seat of the soul, and possibly signs of melancholy, in hearts and other body parts, Burton was more poet than anatomist. In this chapter's epigraph he was writing metaphorically, of course. But more than three hundred years later, Gregory Hemingway would learn that he had inherited, quite literally, a melancholy man's heart. And when Dr. Hemingway's heart failed for the final time in the Miami-Dade Detention Center on October 1, 2001, that heart had been through five decades of a modern version of Burton's "Hell upon earth."

What was melancholy in Burton's time, and what is modern depression? If we need a reminder, and I think we do, the life and the death of Dr. Hemingway remind us that depression is, among other things, a systemic disease, a still-mysterious form of dis-ease that disrupts the mind, the brain, and the body. In this respect depression resembles heart disease, which is also a systemic disease, or more precisely a set of diseases that disrupts many systems.

What is our best current understanding of depression? The capacity of depression to disturb not only our minds but also our social relationships and our most basic physical functioning is hard to escape if you look for it, and yet throughout the wayward history of depression we have frequently lost sight of this systemic view of depression. During most of the twentieth century, for example, the average American, along with mental health clinicians and our leading theorists from Freud to Skinner, viewed depression, even depression as severe as Dr. Hemingway's, as primarily a psychological problem, a disorder of mood. As a practicing psychiatrist for most of the past twenty years, that is how I thought about depression. But now we know with a measure of scientific conviction that depression is more than a problem of mood and the mind.

For young Greg Hemingway, the trouble began early. The third of three boys, he was just nine when his father, Ernest, left his mother for another woman. By the time Greg was fifteen, his father had married four times, including twice more after divorcing Greg's mother, Pauline Pfeiffer Hemingway. At nineteen, Greg got into some trouble that was the subject of a dispute between his parents, a dispute that preceded by hours the death of his mother. When Greg visited his father a few months after the funeral, his father blamed him for her death. Referring to the trouble that led to the dispute, Greg recalled saying to his father, "It wasn't really so bad, Papa." To this Papa said, "No? Well, it killed Mother." Greg believed him. The "yellow-green filter" of depression settled over his mind's eye, he would write later, and it "didn't go away for seven years."[1]

The key elements of his manic-depressive illness had declared themselves by the time he was twenty-three via mood swings, depression, episodic hyperactivity, profligate spending, episodic loss of judgment, and drug and alcohol abuse. Yet, when drafted, he was able to enroll in the army for several years, then finish his premed studies and start medical school. A year into Greg's medical school career, in June 1961, his father rose early one morning in Ketchum, Idaho, leaving his wife, Mary, asleep, put his hunting rifle to his head in the foyer of their home, and pulled the trigger.

"I never got over a sense of responsibility for my father's death," Gregory wrote in *Papa: A Personal Memoir*, "and the recollection of it sometimes made me act in strange ways." To make sense of Gregory Hemingway's depression, it might have sufficed to focus on the psychological impact of the overpowering relationship with his father, because its dynamics say so much about the character of the two men. Gregory's memoir reveals how his usually absent, legendary father remained a dominant force in his life, even many years after his father died. His story of this relationship brings to life the traditional themes of the psychological literature on depression: early childhood loss, death of a parent, unresolved competition with the father, impossible expectations, low self-esteem, identification with the lost parent, anger turned inward, guilt and blame for losses.

But the biology of Dr. Hemingway's depressive illness exerted an influence as powerful as his relationship with his father. And the biology of depression begins with genes. The impact of genes in the Hemingway family is hard to miss. Greg knew that he had inherited "a melancholy man's heart," knew he was the third in a line of three. Second in line was Papa Hemingway, who himself had struggled with mood swings.[2] And though Greg never knew his paternal grandfather, Dr. Clarence Hemingway, he well knew what had happened in Oak Park, Illinois, in 1928. According to Hemingway biographer Michael Reynolds:

> In 1904, Clarence Hemingway took his first self-prescribed rest cure for his "nerves." He suffered similar despondency and irritability in 1907–09 and 1917–19. Each time he moved further into isolation from his family. By 1928, when he put a pistol to his temple and ended his life, he was suffering from diabetes, angina, hypertension, and severe depression—a condition similar to Ernest's own that summer of 1957.[3]

So the sound of his father's shotgun rang out twice for Greg.

Greg inherited his grandfather's illness and pursued his grandfather's profession. If he was at all inclined to deny the lethal nature of his inheritance, his aunt Ursula, Ernest's younger sister, underscored it in 1966 by taking her life with a barbiturate overdose to end her struggle against cancer. In 1982 his uncle Leicester, Ernest's brother, faced with losing his legs to diabetes as his father had, likewise shot himself in the head. And in 1996 Greg's niece, Margaux Hemingway, the daughter of his eldest brother, Jack, like her aunt Ursula, overdosed on barbiturates and died. In spite of requiring multiple treatments for seven episodes of depression, including ninety-seven sessions of electroconvulsive therapy, Gregory Hemingway managed to escape suicide, as did his two brothers. Like his father and his grandfather, by his sixties Gregory had developed high blood pressure and heart disease. He died of congestive heart failure at sixty-nine (see Figure 4.1).[4]

This Hemingway history across four generations drives home the point more tragically than most families that depression, particularly severe

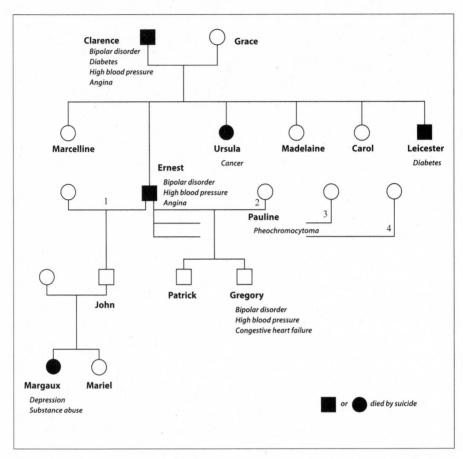

Figure 4.1. Hemingway Family Tree.
This chart illustrates how depression and heart disease can run in families.

depression, runs in families and afflicts the brain and the body, as well as the mind. It afflicts people of average ability, as well as those with creative talent. Among the casualties of depression in his family, only Ernest led a life of extraordinary creative achievement.[5] The Hemingway family history stands out for its pattern of depression and coexisting medical illnesses in midlife: diabetes, high blood pressure, heart disease, cancer. Clarence, Ernest, Leicester, and Gregory Hemingway were each ushered to their ends by the joint forces of depression and cardiovascular disease.

From Black Bile to Genes

What is this mysterious depression? We may experience it as a mood, a character weakness, a waking death, a curse, a disease, or an effective strategy for coping with a loss. Gregory Hemingway experienced it in all these guises. Robert Burton might have experienced it as "black bile." Though clinical depression afflicts all societies, how we think and talk about depression depends on which culture guides us.

A sample of quotations that span seven thousand years and several Western cultures reminds us of what we've known about depression for centuries but have often forgotten.[6] Hippocrates, the patriarch of Western medicine (fifth century B.C.), first described melancholy, *melaina chole*, the black bile, as a humor that afflicts the brain: "It is the brain which makes us mad or delirious, inspires us with dread and fear, whether by night or by day, brings sleeplessness, inopportune mistakes, aimless anxieties, absentmindedness, and acts that are contrary to habit. . . . All these things we endure from the brain, when it is not healthy, but is more hot, more cold, more moist or more dry than natural, or when it suffers any other preternatural or unusual affliction."[7] Melancholia by Hippocrates' definition is the sign of an unhealthy brain. This idea didn't count for much during most of the twentieth century, but now that we know more about the brain it has come to make sense again. Charles Nemeroff, MD, one of the leading current researchers on the relationship between depression and heart disease, has called corticotropin-releasing hormone (CRH), secreted by the brain's hypothalamus, "the black bile of depression."[8]

Galen, an ancient Greek physician (second century A.D.), described patients who experienced "scarce, turbulent, and interrupted sleep, palpitations, vertigo . . . sadness, anxiety, diffidence, and the belief of being persecuted, of being possessed by a demon, hated by the gods. . . . The humor, like a darkness, invades the seat of the soul, where reason is situated. As children who fear the darkness, so adults become when they are the prey of the black bile, which supports fear. For this reason the melancholiacs are afraid of death and wish for it at the same time."[9] Here, Galen was describing the essential physical and psychological elements of what we now call a major depressive episode. This clustering of symptoms has persisted over the ages and is diagnostically useful to us today.

Robert Burton in *The Anatomy of Melancholy* described how depression is a "torment" of both the mind and the body:

> For that which is but a flea-biting to one, causeth insufferable torment to another, & which one by his singular moderation, & well composed carriage can happily overcome, a second is no whit able to sustaine, but upon every small occasion of misconceived abuse, injurie, griefe, disgrace, losse, crosse, rumor, &c. yields so farre to passion, that his complexion is altered, his digestion hindered, his sleepe gone, his spirits obscured, and his heart heavy . . . and he himself overcome with *Melancholy.* . . . If any discontent sease upon a patient, in an instant all other perturbations will set upon him, and then like a lame dogge or broken winged goose hee droopes and pines away, and is brought at last to that malady of melancholy it selfe.[10]

Melancholy is a systemic disease, in Burton's view. In its grip, we droop and pine like lame dogs or broken-winged geese. Depression alters our appearance, our digestion, our sleep, our mood, and our heart.

Hermann Boerhaave, in a 1742 version of the current hypothesis that depression reflects imbalances of neurotransmitters and hormones, proposed that "the brain is a gland and that nervous juices from this gland travel around in the blood. . . . Depression occurs when the oily and fatty stuffs of the blood accumulate and the nervous juices are in short supply."[11] From black bile to nervous juices to serotonin, we refine our ideas about the chemistry of despair.

Clinical Tip 4.1: Think of depression, especially severe depression, as a physical, as well as a psychological and social, illness. This means that once you find trouble in one of these three areas, you ought to see if there are related problems in the other two areas. Is the pain in your back more troublesome when your mood is low? Have disappointments in your family life inflamed your back pain or sapped your strength or scattered your mind so you can't do your job? Closer attention to the physical dimensions sharpens diagnosis of depression and improves the likelihood of its full and effective treatment.

Emil Kraepelin, the pioneering Swiss diagnostician of the late nineteenth and early twentieth century, believed that depression had several causes: "Defective heredity is the most prominent, occurring in from 70 to 80 percent of cases.... Of external causes, beside gestation, alcoholic excesses are the most prominent; others are mental shock, deprivation, and acute diseases."[12] That is, genes, pregnancy, alcohol, stress, poverty, and physical illness all contribute to depression.

Over the centuries, depression has also been called a sin, a personality type, a fashionable philosophy of life, and repressed sadism, to name just a few of our misconceptions. Now we know better.

The Word "Depression"

The word "depression" connotes for some a dip in the economy, for others a dip in the road or a dip in the barometric pressure. For cardiologists the first association of the word depression is often with the ST segment of the electrocardiogram, which is said to be "depressed" during ischemia and heart attacks, as in, "He's got angina, elevated enzymes, and a depressed ST segment" (a sure ticket to the nearest coronary care unit for the owner of that heart).

Depression is a problem too wonderfully complex for a one-word definition. It attacks on so many levels, presents so many faces. And our language hasn't caught up with our understanding.[13] In the United States, the popularization of the psychological use of the word "depression" through movies, the rising use of antidepressant medications over the past decade, the voluminous self-help books on depression (several thousand by one recent count of Barnes and Nobles' titles in print), and the recent political visibility of mental health advocacy groups have both clarified and complicated the use of the term. In the clinical sense of the word that we'll use in this book, at the mild end of the severity spectrum, depression suggests a feeling of sadness, sorrow. This depression is transient and useful, one of the primary colors of our emotional life, along with joy, fear, and anger—a feeling that usually vanishes within minutes or with a good meal or a distracting phone call.

At the severe end of the spectrum lies recurrent major depression, which rarely vanishes with distraction; it's the kind of depression that breaks us and sometimes kills us (see Appendix A). The point along this spectrum of severity where common feeling metastasizes into disabling disorder, where sorrow turns into despair, is a mysterious one. Shifting often, it is peculiar to each of us and to our current circumstances, defined after the event by the intensity and duration of the depression and by how much it disrupted our physical and mental and social functioning. The use of the same word, "depression," to refer to both a sad feeling and a disabling clinical disorder feeds the common misconception that the clinical disorder is all about sadness or excesses of sorrow. In fact, many people with severe clinical depression feel not sad, but numb or irritable or anxious or a confusion of feelings. Profound disruptions of appetite and sleep and libido and physical strength persist in spite of their mood shifts.

In this book I use the word "depression" to refer to a range of clinical depressive disorders, not to the transient sad feeling. These feelings usually take care of themselves, but the disorders keep clinicians like me in business because they slow people down or make them behave in troubling ways that eventually demand help. These depressive disorders include a common set of symptoms or physical signs that impair a person's functioning over a substantial period of time, at least several weeks and often months to years. The average duration of an untreated episode of major depression is four months. These disorders have staying power, and their endurance over many months and sometimes years exacts a toll on the heart.

The American Psychiatric Association and the International Classification of Diseases classify depression as a mood disorder, as opposed to a thought disorder or an anxiety disorder.[14] These terms, with their emphasis on a particular symptom, signal an arbitrary convenience of classification more than an overriding fact about the primary importance of mood or thought or anxiety for any particular disorder. Just as schizophrenia is more than disordered thought, depression is more than disordered mood. Though each has its distinctive pattern, both disorders wreak havoc on mood, thought, and sense of well-being, to say nothing of the body.

Dr. Henry Maudsley, a nineteenth-century English psychiatrist, called depression "a profound pain of mind paralyzing its functions."[15] The phrase "pain of mind" should guide us. It helps to think of depression as a pain syndrome, the way we think of physical pain, like chest pain, and the way we thought of the syndrome of heart disease a hundred years ago, before we understood its many causes and pathologies. I've been referring to clinical depression as a "disease" in the loose sense of the term. More precisely, depression is a syndrome, a collection of symptoms and behaviors, as opposed to a single disease (like coronary disease, with proven causes and pathophysiologies).

But a syndrome does not tell us about the biological, psychological, or social mechanisms that produced the symptoms. Just as a chest-pain syndrome (sharp pains, lightheadedness, sweating, and fatigue) in four different people may be the work of either hardened arteries, a burning ulcer in the esophagus, an infection in the pericardial sac, or a blood clot in the lung, many factors and pathways may contribute to the syndrome of a depressive episode.

Clinical Tip 4.2: Chart the course of your depression over your lifetime. Have you ever tried to draw a picture of the number of days, weeks, or months in your lifetime when you have been clinically depressed? It's a useful exercise because it shows you something you probably didn't understand about the duration or severity of your depression. Most of us avoid thinking quantitatively about something as experiential and painful as depression. How many episodes of moderate or severe depression have you had? How long did they last? Did you recover fully or only partially? See Appendix B, "Charting the Course of Depression," for examples and guidelines on how to chart your depression. Try it, and discuss your chart with selected supportive members of your family and your doctor. If you have had two or more episodes of major depression, your risk for developing heart disease is greater than if you have had only one episode or more mild symptoms. And if you already have coronary disease, the importance of treating the depressive episodes is greater if you've had two or more episodes of depression than if you are experiencing your first.[16]

We now recognize several types of depression based on symptoms, course, biology, and family history, and we're only beginning to understand the possible causes and pathologic mechanisms for these various types. Once we understand the pathology of mental illnesses in biologic terms (not next year, but maybe in a decade or two), the diagnostic classification of depressive disorders will undergo a radical revision and the terms will change. Until then, the current terms are worth understanding because, since their introduction around 1980, they have provided an international vocabulary for research and treatment advances, as well as for books on depression for the general public. (If you are unfamiliar with the types of depression and the diagnostic terms, see Appendix C, "Types of Depression"; for a discussion of the assessment of depression, see Appendix D, "Assessment of Depression.")

The Psychological Effects of Depression

Depression is often about losses, external losses as well as perceived ones.[17] The most severe depressions shut down our most basic mental functions, such as thought and speech and perception—leaving us in what Maudsley called mental paralysis. Before Greg Hemingway reached twenty, he had faced at least two big losses, the loss of his father to divorce and the loss of his mother to death. Longitudinal studies of children who lose a parent to death, separation, or illness show that early losses raise one's chances of depression in adulthood. And losses as an adult add to the burden of depression. A large Danish epidemiologic study recently reported that parents who lost a child to death suffered increased rates of heart attacks up to seventeen years later, with sudden infant deaths causing the greatest rise in parental depression rates.[18]

The psychology of depression may derail the best efforts of people with heart disease to manage their illness. The loss of hope, the infamous pessimism of depression, may make the complex cardiac rehabilitation treatment plans appear futile. The limited concentration and capacity to reason that come with many depressions may make a complex regimen (such as: six white pills three times a day, two pink pills twice a day, exercise three times a week, low-salt diet every meal, and don't argue with your boss) feel frustrating or overwhelming. Managing heart disease is a challenging, long haul for anyone, and depressed patients give up sooner than most.

Low self-esteem differentiates clinical depression from bereavement. Bereavement by itself does not lower our opinion of ourselves, but Gregory Hemingway's grief over his mother's death soon developed into a clinical depression that resulted in his dropping out of college, doubting that he could become a doctor. When the low self-esteem of depression meets the job loss or loss of physical vigor that follows a heart attack or repeated bouts of chest pain, the result can be psychologically devastating. The heart disease appears to confirm the self-doubt, and the depression in turn magnifies the impairments of the heart disease. Depressed patients report more chest pain and take longer to return to work after a heart attack.

William Styron, acclaimed author of *Sophie's Choice* and five other novels, wrote about his experience of loss during depression in *Darkness Visible: A Memoir of Madness*:

> Much obviously remains to be learned . . . , but certainly one psychological element has been established beyond reasonable doubt, and that is the concept of loss. Loss in all of its manifestations is the touchstone of depression—in the progress of the disease and, most likely, in its origin. At a later date I would gradually be persuaded that devastating loss in childhood figured as a probable genesis of my own disorder; meanwhile, as I monitored my retrograde condition, I felt loss at every hand. The loss of self-esteem is a celebrated symptom, and my own sense of self had all but disappeared, along with any self-reliance. This loss can quickly degenerate into dependence, and from dependence into infantile dread. One dreads the loss of all things, all people close and dear. There is an acute fear of abandonment. Being alone in the house, even for a moment, caused me exquisite panic and trepidation.[19]

Depression is about losses, including loss of control. In the mid-twentieth century, the behaviorists, led by B. F. Skinner, who scoffed at all the untestable psychoanalytic speculations, responded with a model for depression called "learned helplessness." Martin Seligman at the University of Pennsylvania and others developed animal models of learned helplessness that approximate some features of human depression. Rats exposed to electrical shocks in cages with no escape or control over the shocks soon lay down and suffered their pains without resistance, their hearts racing and their appetites deadened and their interest in their surroundings shut down. Monkeys respond the same way. So do some humans in laboratory conditions and jails and sometimes in hospitals. As George Engel has pointed out, in settings where the perception of loss of control accurately reflects one's options, conservation-withdrawal provides an adaptive response to an impossible situation.[20] Confinement in an intensive care unit after a heart attack forces a state of relative helplessness on people who are used to controlling their daily lives. For brief periods of time in such settings, relinquishing control or acting helpless may be adaptive and hasten recovery.

However, depression fails to be adaptive when the perception of loss of control denies the available options, that is, when we perceive ourselves to be more helpless than we are. We misread our situation. Our judgment fails us. Depression is also about loss of judgment and reason and the misinterpretation of information. In the 1950s, when most psychoanalysts and behaviorists in the United States would not talk to each other, Aaron Beck, a psychiatrist with psychoanalytic training who dared to learn from the behaviorists, first described in modern clinical terms the patterns of dysfunctional thinking so characteristic of the depressed mind. He described the cognitive triad of negative thoughts about oneself, one's past, and the future that dominate during a depressive episode. To identify with this outlook, think of the brooding, the morbid ruminations, and the pessimistic predictions that cloud your darkest moods.

To explain how dysfunctional thoughts contribute to depression, Beck developed the cognitive model of depression, which proposed that stressful situations trigger automatic thoughts or lightning-fast appraisals of a situation, similar to the subconscious free associations described by psychoanalysis. In the depressed mind the dominant negative automatic thoughts lead to depressed feelings and helpless behaviors. Underlying depressive schemas or beliefs about the way the world works drive the selection of automatic thoughts. During depression, the dormant schemas, developed at times of previous losses or failures and tucked away in the attics of our minds, jump into action and dominate our appraisal of stressful situations, coloring them dark.[21] Beck translated into a practical theory for the treatment of depression what Aretaeus observed several thousand years ago about the cognitive distortions of depression: "The melancholic isolates himself; he is afraid of being persecuted and imprisoned; he torments himself with superstitious ideas; he is terror-stricken; he mistakes his fantasies for the truth; he complains of imaginary diseases; he curses life and wishes for death."[22]

Beck observed that depressed people could learn to modify these distortions in a matter of weeks to a few months, and by practicing more adaptive ways of thinking they could achieve relief from depression, even from severe depression. This observation revolutionized the psychotherapy of depression.

The Social Effects of Depression

Some experts have argued that depression is primarily a social problem, a sign of faulty relationships. Social relationships have the power to inflict depression on us and the power to protect us from depression. Gregory Hemingway went to visit his father after the death of his mother, hoping for relief from his grief. Instead he met with blame, which he felt fixed the "yellow-green filter" of depression upon him for the next seven years. Andrew Solomon, who experienced severe depression numerous times, also for the first time after the death of his mother, opens *The Noonday Demon*, his five-hundred-page memoir and essay on depression, with these lines: "Depression is the flaw in love. To be creatures who love, we must be creatures who can despair at what we lose, and depression is the mechanism of that despair."

Despair is contagious. We are wired to sense the moods of others, especially depression. Entering the room of a person with severe depression is a visceral, almost contagious experience, like sensing a pungent odor. Why are we so sensitive to depression in others? Evolutionary psychology has proposed that a capacity for depression serves a useful purpose for some social groups. Depression has survived as a universal trait in all cultures of our species. Because most species and all primates survive longer and reproduce more efficiently in groups than alone, natural selection has favored traits that promote the social functions of the species, particularly the functioning of small groups such as nuclear families, extended families, neighborhoods or villages, and tribes. At each of these levels of social organization, the establishment of hierarchies favors the survival of the group. Competition for power at every level of the hierarchy creates winners and losers. The submissive response of the loser (slouching posture, withdrawal, silence, loss of aggression) promotes the winner's capacity to lead the group. A loser who refuses to submit and retreat interferes with the leader's exercise of power.[23]

This argument for the adaptive value of a capacity for depression applies to our modern industrial society, where we spar for power with words instead of weapons, usually. If we did not suffer depression after the loss of rank or social role or close relationships, we'd be less careful about our attachments, less caring about each other. Except for the sociopaths with no conscience, who require other forms of punishment, nature punishes social neglect and social isolation with depression. Depressed behaviors also function to communicate one's need for help, often eliciting a rallying response from close friends. And depression forces disengagement from futile tasks, conserving resources for other, more productive tasks. It can be good to feel bad.

Poverty may be the most striking social dimension of chronic depression. In the United States, poor people experience roughly double the rates of depression of middle- and upper-class groups. In one recent report the rates of current major depression among the poor ranged from 16 to 30 percent, three times the rate in the general population. Rates of depression among people on Medicaid range from 30 to 50 percent, and one recent study found depression in 53 percent of pregnant women on Medicaid.[24]

Does poverty make people depressed, or does depression make people poor? Look at the personal and family histories of the depressed poor. Depression causes more days missed from work in the United States than do other common chronic conditions, such as heart disease, diabetes, hypertension, or back pain. When depression persists for months to years, it costs people their jobs. Loss of a job in the United States usually means loss of health insurance along with loss of income. If depression makes you lose your job, you've also lost your access to the treatment that would relieve you of this problem. So the downward spiral begins.[25]

How do the social dimensions of depression relate to heart disease? James J. Lynch, a physiological psychologist at the University of Maryland, devoted his career to studying the effects of social contact on the cardiovascular system. His first book, *The Broken Heart: The Medical Consequences of Loneliness*, published in 1977, described the impact of various forms of social isolation on heart disease rates in the United States. He pointed to the rising divorce rates and identified a pattern of substantially higher rates among the divorced compared to the married from all causes of premature death among adults between twenty-four and sixty-five, led by cardiovascular deaths. Similar trends held for the single, widowed, and separated, and these demographic facts about cardiovascular mortality risk and social isolation remain true today.

Lynch looked at Utah to exemplify the social dimensions of heart disease. In the 1960s Utah had one of the lowest premature death rates in the country, whereas neighboring Nevada, comparable in average annual income, education level, proportion of city dwellers, number of citizens, and doctors and hospitals, led the country in premature death rates, including cardiovascular deaths. Lynch attributed the difference in death rates to the dramatic differences in divorce rates, mobility, and religious tradition between the populations of these two states. Utah had half the divorce rate of Nevada, and more than 60 percent of the state's adults had been born there. In Nevada 90 percent of its citizens were born someplace else, and residential moves in and out of the state were common. Utah's Mormon heritage anchored its families to their home state and the church community, with apparent good effects for their hearts.

When social isolation and depression occur together, as they often do, it's bad for the heart. Bereavement among the elderly increases the rate of death by heart disease for the next six to twelve months, after which the rate returns to normal. The rate of suicide among spouses also increases during the first year of bereavement and then diminishes. Nancy Frasure-Smith, a sociologist and professor of psychiatry at McGill University and a leading investigator in the study of depression and heart disease, found that high levels of depression following a heart attack predict early death by heart disease within the next the next six to eighteen months. However, she also found that high levels of social support buffer the impact of depression on these death rates. That is, strong social ties help relieve depressive symptoms faster and protect against the higher risk of dying from heart disease. Women with satisfying marriages, compared to single women and those with unsatisfying marriages, have less atherosclerosis in their hearts. Love can buffer your heart from the ravages of your mind.[26]

In his second book, *The Language of the Heart: The Body's Response to Human Dialogue,* Lynch described the exquisite sensitivity of the cardiovascular system to conversation, touch, and communication in general.[27] Communication may raise or lower blood pressure, depending on how demanding or reassuring it is. People with high resting blood pressure tend to react to communication with greater increases in blood pressure than do people with normal blood pressure when the talk demands too much of them. Heart rate and rhythm, and our ability to vary them, may improve or worsen with dialogue. Recent studies have shown that depression tends to reduce heart rate variability (HRV), which is a bad thing, because hearts work best when they can vary their rates in response to demands. Hearts that can't vary their rates die more easily, and reduced HRV predicts reduced survival in people with coronary disease.[28]

These studies all preach the same lesson: Social isolation is bad for heart disease. Anything that contributes to social isolation as forcefully as depression does will worsen heart disease.[29]

Clinical Tip 4.3: Count your social supports. Because both depression and heart disease are profoundly influenced by social factors, it's important to take stock of whom you can turn to for help with each of these problems. How many people close to you know about your heart disease? How helpful are they? How many people close to you know about your depression? How helpful are they? Most people with either of these illnesses need an informal team of at least several people from among family and friends with whom they can talk, share resources, and learn practical knowledge. Make sure they know you're counting on them. If you don't have a supportive team, talk to your doctor about how to build one.

Though social factors play powerful roles in the course of depression, it's too simplistic to say, as Thomas Szasz argued in *The Myth of Mental Illness* (1960), that depression is fundamentally a social problem. Most poor people manage to avoid clinical depression. More often than not we adapt to interpersonal losses without requiring treatment for depression. And depression occurs around the world in fairly consistent numbers in spite of wide variations in social conditions. The argument for the importance of social factors applies to many chronic illnesses. For example, social isolation, cultural habits of diet and exercise, and poverty play powerful roles in determining the course of heart disease. The more compelling view, one that fits the epidemiology and the personal histories of most people with depression, argues that depression begins in the mind, brain, and body, then spawns or amplifies social problems, which in turn contribute to depression. By the time we see the illness, the psychological and the social factors have been playing on the biological factors for months to years, sometimes for generations, and it's hard to uncover what got the process started.

The Physical Effects of Depression

Since Hippocrates intuited that melancholy originated in the brain, we have either taken his assertion on faith or disputed it, but the biology underlying the physical effects of depression has remained a mystery to all but the most visionary researchers in the field. In the last half of the twentieth century, however, the pieces of a biological picture of depression have emerged: the neuroanatomy of the emotional brain, the chemistry of neurotransmitters, the physiology of the neuron and the synapse, the molecular biology of genes in depression. These findings put into a biological context what we have long known about the failings of the depressed mind. But only in the last ten years have the pieces begun to come together in a coherent picture of the broad outlines of the neurobiology of depression. Much remains unknown, but now we can describe the essentials of the anatomy, chemistry, physiology, and genetics of depression. And the picture argues persuasively for Hippocrates' guess that depression begins in the brain, specifically the emotional brain or the limbic system, and disrupts other systems in the body, including the circulatory system.

That does not mean that depression is no longer a problem of the mind. The mind is where we live depression, where we can't avoid it. We can't see or sense the brain except though the mind. Understanding the psychology of depression helps us as far as it goes, but until we understand the workings of the brain and the body during all phases of depression, this clinical disorder will remain just a fascinating and terrifying mystery of the mind.

Our bodies work differently when we're depressed, especially when we're severely depressed. Depression can disrupt our hormones (ACTH, cortisol), our inflammatory system (cytokines) in the heart and brain, and our bones, as well as our hearts (increased sympathetic outflow), as Figure 4.2 shows. We get fat in funny ways, mostly in the adipose tissue of the belly, and our bones grow thinner because of excess cortisol. Our most basic physical functions, such as sleep, appetite, sex, and pain sensation, slip

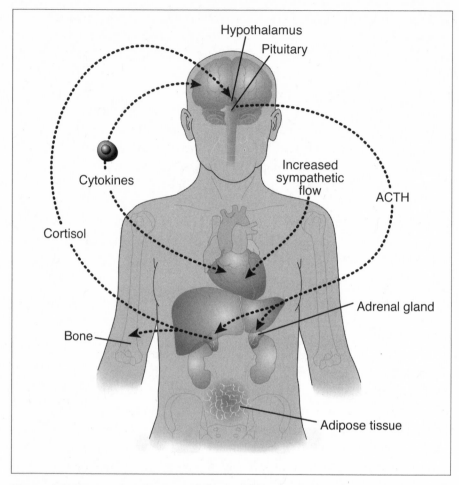

Figure 4.2. Depression: Disease of the Mind, Brain, and Body.
Depression can dysregulate hormones, inflammation, and bone strength.
Source: modified from Gold 2002a.

out of synch. Most people who have been through a depressive episode can tell you at least one way in which their bodies felt odd or out of synch. William Styron's gait and voice changed:

> The normal circuits began to drown, causing some of the functions of the body and nearly all of those of instinct and intellect to slowly disconnect. . . . I particularly remember the lamentable near disappear-

ance of my voice. It underwent a strange transformation, becoming at times quite faint, wheezy and spasmodic—a friend observed later that it was the voice of a ninety-year-old. The libido also made an early exit, as it does in most major illnesses—it is the superfluous need of a body in beleaguered emergency. Many people lose all appetite; mine was relatively normal, but I found myself eating only for subsistence: food, like everything else within the scope of sensation, was utterly without savor. Most distressing of all the instinctual disruptions was that of sleep, along with a complete absence of dreams. Exhaustion combined with sleeplessness is a rare torture.[30]

The face sags, the shoulders droop, the hand hesitates. The chef loses his sense of taste. Dancers lose their rhythm. The architecture of the sleep cycle collapses. Laborers tire quicker and rest longer. Physical fatigue sets in early in the day, without explanation, and often persists to the point of exhaustion.[31] Pain is amplified, also without explanation. Handwriting turns unsteady or the spoon rattles against the coffee cup. Some people tolerate these effects as inconveniences. Others are overwhelmed by them.

Depression causes more *physical* disability and keeps more people in bed each month than does back pain, arthritis, or lung disease. The days lost from work reflect the physical distress of depression as much as the mental distress. The only common chronic illness that causes more physical disability than depression is coronary disease.[32]

It's easy to confuse depression with physical illness. The first few days of most physical illnesses, whether it's the flu or a fracture or an inflamed joint, bring with them the generic manifestations of depression: low mood, fatigue, social withdrawal, loss of appetite, sluggish thinking. These changes may be adaptive if they are brief and timed with the onset of the physical illness. Depression shares with many physical illnesses this conservation-withdrawal syndrome, which helps us put off the rest of life, withdrawing and conserving while we manage the physical insult. However, underneath its emotional and mental disturbances, persistent clinical depression shares many of the systemic biologic changes that occur in acute physical illnesses. As we'll see in the next chapter, circulating cytokines from the inflamed coronary arteries may have a direct depressive effect on the central nervous system.

Some women get a monthly visit from this set of depressive symptoms as part of a premenstrual syndrome. It feels like a scheduled bout with depression, every thirty days. Sudden shifts in estrogen and progesterone at the end of a period, a pregnancy, or menopause can mimic the depressions that come at other times—powerful evidence for one of the physical dimensions of depression.

Clinical Tip 4.4: Know the physical dimensions of your depression. If your depression is severe enough to require treatment with either medications or psychotherapy, get a good physical exam from a doctor who can help you understand the physical dimensions of your depression. Good primary care doctors and many specialists will talk to you about the physical dimensions of your depression. Keep a list of the physical problems that develop with each depressive episode. These physical characteristics of depression may be useful to you as warning signs of future depressions or as symptoms that need to be resolved to achieve full recovery from the current depression. How much of your fatigue, pain, weakness, nausea, tremors, or any other combination of symptoms is attributable to depression? How much to heart disease? Sometimes these questions can be answered only by trying specific treatments and seeing which symptoms improve. For example, if you have high blood pressure, what does effective treatment of your depression do for your high blood pressure?

Depression interferes with the course of physical illnesses as varied as coronary disease, diabetes, AIDS, and hepatitis, illnesses whose pathology occurs in organ systems well removed from the mind and the brain. How can a mood disorder muck up the workings of the heart in one person, the pancreas in another, and in another the immune system or the liver? The answer, in the words of one international expert on depression, A. John Rush, MD, of the University of Texas Southwestern, is that "the brain is the organ of the mind."[33] A disturbed brain presents itself as a disturbed mind. And the brain has a long reach, as we shall see. It extends to everywhere in the body. Disturb the brain for long, and the brain disturbs the body.

CHAPTER 5

Depression and the Biology Window

A feeling is the momentary "view" of a part
of that body landscape.
—Antonio Damasio, *Descartes' Error*

Gloria Wachuka at fifty-two is a defiantly cheerful woman with a quick laugh and a faith that has deepened through her long experience with depression. Nothing in her voice or her face or her posture hints at her thirty years of grappling with the darker side of her nature. Her garden and living room are crowded with statuettes, dolls, and angels she has made, icons of good cheer which over the past few years she has sold as a hobby. Now, as she talks of her worst depression ten years ago, just a year after her heart attack at thirty-eight, she smiles and chuckles nervously about what a different woman she was during those six months. Her voice is full and strong.

> I didn't eat during that time. Usually when I'm down I eat. Nervous eating, you know, cakes, cookies, candy, ice cream, all that delicious, nasty stuff. Not this time. I didn't want any of that. I just shut myself in. I wouldn't go out. Shut myself away from friends, shut myself away from work. I couldn't tell you why. I was just afraid something bad would happen and I didn't know what. Seemed like I just couldn't get myself out the door. That's all there was to it and that's not me. Normally I was running around with my head cut off chasing the kids this way and that. But this time I couldn't do that. I lost my phlebotomy job at the hospital and couldn't ask for disability, couldn't face that, so I was off work six months. All I could think about day and night for

months was how mad I was at my youngest daughter's father for how bad he treated her way back when she was little. It was unbearable.

That time changed me. I really think some of my friends didn't recognize me, you know, when I called on the phone, like they didn't recognize my voice at first. Two of my friends asked me if I was coming down with something, bronchitis maybe, because I sounded so thin and shaky. One friend I worked with for two years at the hospital, I swear she didn't recognize me when I ran into her at the crafts store. I didn't know I looked any different. She couldn't even come up with my name, like I'd shocked her. I just went home and cried and looked at my face in the bathroom mirror and maybe it did look like somebody else's face and I prayed, Lord, what has become of me?

More than once Gloria thought about suicide, but she'd seen a young girl in the neighborhood lose her mother to suicide, and she couldn't do that to her three. Where was her faith? It was so hard to pray. "They told me I had what they call a chemical imbalance. Well, I guess so, but it was something else. . . . Never, never again. Every day I pray never again."

Feelings as Windows

What was Gloria's "chemical imbalance"? What was going on in her brain and her body during those six months of the worst depression of her life? We often think of feelings as windows to the mind, but feelings are also windows to the brain and the body, as Antonio Damasio wrote in *Descartes' Error*. And we are beginning to see how the biology of depression merges with the biology of heart disease. What is the chemistry of a half-dead mind? Why couldn't Gloria move herself to get out of the house and go to work? How did the changes in her brain from depression affect the changes in her heart disease?

These are now exciting and promising questions, but searching for the biology of depression, or the biology of any mental illness, for that matter, was an unfashionable, unrewarding business for most of the twentieth century. Few pursued it. Until the 1960s, no one had proposed a sound argument for depression's being a brain disorder. And until the past ten years, it wasn't clear whether the answers would be found in anatomic brain pathways, the chemistry of neurotransmitters, intracellular chemistry, or possibly genes. Early efforts to identify brain structures and defective physiological processes that were specific to depression frustrated many investigators and kept the cloak of mystery tightly wrapped around depression.

But as the tools for studying the brain proliferated—from chemical probes for dissecting the synapses to imaging scans for charting the active brain—the windows began to open on the whole central nervous system. Investigators studying the neurobiology of depression have found disruptions in all levels of the nervous system: the anatomy of the emotional brain, the neural regulation of stress hormones and the heart, and the neurotransmitters of the brain—and, of course, at the level of our genes. Psychiatrist Eric Kandel won the Nobel Prize in medicine in 2000 for his work on the genetic and intracellular processes of brain cells that drive learning and memory, many of which go awry during depression.[1]

It is no longer defensible to deny that major depression is a brain disorder, as well as an illness. Precisely how this brain disorder works remains to be spelled out in detail. We now know the major pieces of the puzzle, but not yet exactly how they fit together. One set of pieces that has recently come together shows how feelings represent physical states. Neurologist Antonio Damasio, in *Descartes' Error*, has described the complex patterns of physiological states that we call the many shades of anger, joy, sadness, and fear. Imagine the number of patterns of muscle tension in the face. Add the variations in body posture. Combine these with rises or falls in heart rate, skin resistance, gastric secretion, sphincter tone, body temperature—most of which we never notice.[2] These patterns register in our minds as feelings, sometimes too subtle for words, sometimes stark and simple. As we grow up, we give the simpler feelings names. Often our names for these feelings are clumsy—"love" and "rage" are too generic to express the subtle variations of what we often feel. Feeling names in most languages don't capture the subtleties of the pattern, don't imply at all which body parts are affected or how. Most of us remain in the dark about the physicality of our feelings, but feelings, as Damasio tells us, are windows into the body. Neuroscientists are just now learning how to look through those windows. Depression, both as a feeling and as a disorder, gives us a window into the interior body.

Many biological mechanisms contribute to depression, but one set of neuroendocrine mechanisms for depression relates to the biology of heart disease. In Chapters 2 and 3 we looked at the scientific background for the behavioral pathway from depression to heart disease. In this and the next chapter we'll look at the background for the biological pathway: the dys-regulations of the limbic system and the stress-response system that form the essential features of the neuroendocrine pathway between depression and heart disease.

Rather than viewing Gloria's heart attack at thirty-eight as a fluke or just bad heart genes, it makes more sense, and it's more useful, to view her heart attack in the context of the biology of the depression that preceded and followed it. To understand how the brain breaks down under stress and depression, and how it affects heart disease, we need a crash course in a few aspects of brain anatomy, a few key neural circuits, the brain chemistry of depression, and a bit about genes that control the growth of nerves in the brain.

Snapshots of the Three Brains

Picture the brain. To the naked and uninitiated eye the brain looks about as impressive as a well-cooked cauliflower—just as mushy, but grayer, more rumpled, more slippery, and smaller than our vanity would like it to be. If you could stand the sensation, a human brain could sit comfortably in one of your hands, just two grayish hemispheres and a stump. The brain's hemispheres appear to have been crammed into a bowl two sizes too small. If you slip your thumbs in between the hemispheres, and pull them apart, the inside gives you more gray and some streaks of white and a few pockets and creases here and there, but it's not obvious at first that you're holding three brains and an organ with many parts. It still looks like a cauliflower.[3]

The three brains, as Figure 5.1 shows, are the primitive brain, the emotional brain, and the new brain. The most primitive, instinctive, or "reptilian" brain, which coordinates our more automatic functions such as heart rate, blood pressure, breathing, pain signals, muscle coordination, and reflexes, sits in the lowest and oldest (evolutionarily speaking) part of the brain, the brainstem. The cerebellum is a mini-brain, a cauliflowerette that hangs off the back of the brainstem, wedged under the hind end of the hemispheres. The cerebellum is part of the primitive brain. Without the primitive brain you die, fast.

The next phase in the evolution of the brain came with the mammals

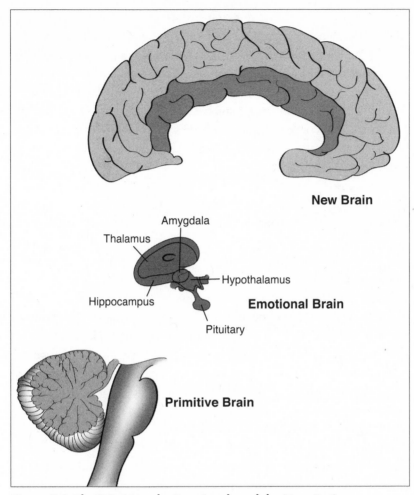

Figure 5.1. The Primitive, the Emotional, and the New Brain

and the emergence of the emotional brain, which wraps over the top of the brainstem like a hand palming a walking stick. Anatomists often call this collection of structures the limbic system. Rats and everything superior to rats have limbic systems, but snails don't. Without this emotional brain, we mammals act odd for a while, very odd, and then we die. Regulation of emotions turns out to be crucial to our survival, crucial to the survival of any complex mammal, even the ones we think of as short on feelings, like gophers and aardvarks. And this regulation of emotions requires a delicate synchrony of many structures and networks within the limbic system.

The limbic system synthesizes information about sensations from our bodies and our environment (pain, sights, odors, etc.) and links the sensations to memories and conscious thought. Through a variety of circuits, the limbic system assembles the complex emotional constructs we call fear and joy and sadness and communicates these emotions to the cortex, where reason tries to make sense of the signals and guide our response. (When I hear a rattle in the grass, do I run, shout, or smile?) In this way the limbic system mediates between sensory information coming in from below through the brainstem and our more advanced capacities for reason and consciousness coming down from above, in an effort to make sense of our place in our environment.[4]

Over the emotional brain and the limbic system, evolution gradually wrapped the new brain, the neocortex. Its cerebral hemispheres house the executive functions, such as attention and complex learning and, in humans, speech and reasoning and conscious thought and some forms of memory and a sense of humor. The cortex of the cerebral hemispheres orchestrates much of the action below, mostly by constraining or harnessing the mammalian emotions of the limbic system into something more human. We can live without our cerebral hemispheres. Not fun or pretty or humane, but possible. So the neocortex wraps around the limbic system which wraps around the brainstem. The human constrains the mammal, which constrains the reptile in us.

Understanding the biology of depression begins with understanding how the limbic system communicates and miscommunicates with the cortex. What was going awry in Gloria's limbic system and her cortex that made her feel and function so differently for those six months at age thirty-nine? The parts of the cortex that play important roles in depression lie mostly up front in the regions that serve attention, motivation, and the regulation of thoughts and feelings. The most important areas, shown in Figure 5.2, include the prefrontal cortex, which lies in the front end above the eyes and around the side near the temple, and the anterior cingulate cortex, which lies deeper and runs along the midline over the corpus callosum, the bridge between the two hemispheres.

During a major depressive episode, these areas of the brain are—liter-

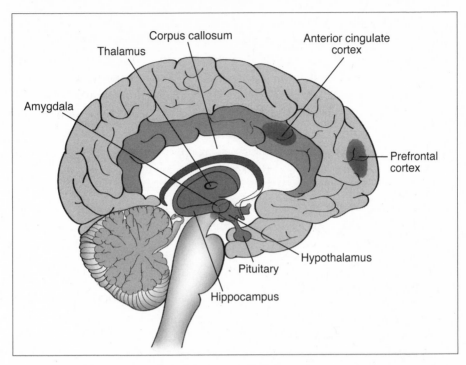

Figure 5.2. The Cortex and Limbic System in Depression

ally—depressed. They don't function at their usual levels of activity. Gloria finds it a struggle to pray, to pay attention at her job, to work up the stuff to motivate herself to do what she usually does without thinking twice about it. Simple routines become complex, overwhelming tasks. Keeping control of her thoughts and feelings, usually so automatic, now eludes her. She reverts to ruminating over old wounds, and the pain at times rises to "unbearable." She had no brain scan at the time, but now it is possible to demonstrate in people with depressions like hers that the cells in the prefrontal cortex and the anterior cingulate areas are less active than they should be. During the depressive episode these areas consume less glucose, the major fuel for brain cells. They return to normal activity when the depression resolves.[5]

Gloria's prefrontal cortex, like yours and mine, is in charge of estimating rewards and punishments in threatening situations, shifting emotions to adapt to new situations, and facilitating complex cognitive processes.

Sophisticated stuff, and the sort of action she needs when navigating a delicate job like drawing blood from patients, falling in love with a man, or managing three kids' daily lives as a single mother. The prefrontal cortex also keeps a tight hand on the amygdala and the hypothalamus, restraining these areas from overreacting to stress. Gloria needed her prefrontal cortex to be sharp. When it turned dull and depressed, she felt it, and it showed.

The cingulate gyrus (see the darkly shaded area in Figure 5.2), from its position between the limbic system and the centers of higher thought, regulates the blending of thoughts and feelings, and so gives meaning to the flow of information in our daily lives. Injury or decreased activity in anterior cingulate area leads to that sense of meaninglessness that robs us of pleasure, hope, and, for some, the will to live. From the depths of her depression, Gloria saw her life as flat, dead, meaningless—to her and, she felt, to God.

The Loopy Limbic System

When these areas of the cortex are depressed, the limbic system below them reacts. The key structures of the limbic system, the emotional brain, are pictured in Figure 5.2. The thalamus, the hypothalamus, the hippocampus, and the amygdala are the areas most relevant to depression. All these structures of the limbic system are packed into an area smaller than a baby's fist. Instead of being dampened down, as is the cortex, these parts of the limbic system are often turned up during severe depression, overly active and reactive.

The thalamus is our relay station. It sits like a chestnut near the top and center of the limbic system, receiving and sorting all incoming sensory information, such as signals from the eyes and ears, the skin, the heart, the spinal cord. Just under the thalamus is the hypothalamus, the central coordinator of our most basic drives, such as appetite, sleep, the stress response, and the sexual response. Below the hypothalamus hangs the pituitary, the pea-sized source of our hormones for regulating the stress response and the sexual response, as well as processes as varied as growth rates, metabolic rate, and the balance of salt and water.

The thalamus relay station sends out information relevant to emotion along two pathways: (1) a short loop down to the hypothalamus, then out to the amygdala and hippocampus on each side; and (2) a long loop up and forward to the cortex. The older, shorter, and faster loop to the almond-shaped amygdala is designed for reflex actions, such as fleeing danger or smiling with affection. The central part of the amygdala directly connects by nerve fibers to the centers in the brainstem that control heart rate, so it can jumpstart the heart as fast as a nerve impulse can travel. The amygdala has a memory of sorts, a limited library of reflex responses to send out to the motor and hormonal systems. Here, then, is one of the most primitive links between the emotional brain and the heart—through the amygdala, the emotional reflex responder.

Next to the amygdala on each side and tightly connected to it, the hippocampus houses a larger library of emotional memories with which it turns the response of the amygdala down or up, for a more finely tuned reaction. So the hippocampus's main function is to adjust or modify the automatic responses of the amygdala.

Another modifying influence on the amygdala is the longer, slower, but more sophisticated loop that runs from the thalamus up to the prefrontal

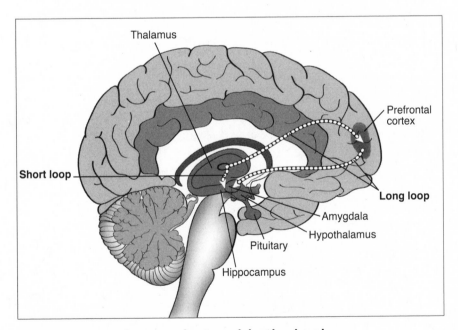

Figure 5.3. Two Pathways to the Amygdala. The short loop carries the reflex responses of the amygdala; the longer loop allows more sophisticated responses and restraint.

cortex and back down to the amygdala. This loop brings reason and more complex memory and learning to bear on the amygdala—sometimes snuffing out all action, other times consciously selecting a different response than the amygdala by itself would have delivered. When this longer loop dominates, will power overrules instinct, and civilized behavior restrains impulsive behavior.[6]

How does this emotional brain work during depression? Not well, of course, and the effect is sometimes loopy. The conductor has walked out on the orchestra, and parts of the depressed brain play too hard while others play not hard enough. They're off-key and out of synch. One overarching finding that has emerged in brain-imaging studies of depressed patients is a pattern of decreased activity in key areas of the cortex, coupled with a pattern of increased activity in key areas of the limbic system. It's not the whole brain that is depressed, but specific parts of the cortex: the prefrontal cortex, the anterior cingulate cortex, and the inferior parietal region. Helen Mayberg, MD, associate professor of neurology at the University of Toronto, has shown how an area of the anterior cingulate cortex called CG24a shows low metabolic activity during depression, then increases its metabolic activity during the process of recovering from depression. Other studies have shown similar improvements in underactive cortical areas during response to treatment.[7]

But the picture of the brain with a few of its lights out doesn't capture the torment of depression. While crucial cortical areas slog along, barely showing any activity, other mostly deeper brain structures are firing without restraint, particularly in the limbic system. The middle part of the thalamus relay station works overtime, sending too many signals to the parts of the amygdala that reflexively respond to distress. The resulting overactivity in the amygdala generates the anxiety and the emotional fragility that so commonly riddle depression. Gloria's overactive limbic system shut her inside her house, showering her with signals of threat that made no sense to her, and sapped her of her courage and faith and energy.[8]

The important picture emerging now from these brain-imaging studies is that depression reflects a shift in the delicate balance of activity between the limbic system and the higher functions of the cortex, a shift that tips too much in favor of a poorly regulated limbic system.[9] In this sense, Gloria Wachuka's depression is an electrical imbalance as well as a chemical imbalance. Rather than looking only at brain chemistry, as earlier theories have, this model for describing the biology of depression focuses on the anatomy of the emotional brain, the circuits that connect its structures to the cortex, and the many ways to regulate these circuits. When the cortical regulation over the limbic system slips, tires out, or fails, we lose our finely tuned control over our emotions, our thinking, and our daily rhythms. No wonder we act loopy. The many possible ways for this complex system to fail may account for the many possible combinations of features of depression. Some depressed people feel anxious, jittery, and can't sleep, while others feel like lead, sleep fourteen hours a night, and wake up exhausted. Some stay depressed for years, others only for weeks. Some develop heart disease, others don't.

The Faulty Stress-Response System

Survival, in the evolutionary sense, demands resilience and the ability to maintain stability in spite of environmental change. Humans have evolved the most elaborate system for responding to the challenges of weather, combat, hunger, crowding, disease, and even the hassles of heavy traffic. The key to the effectiveness of this stress-response system is the seemingly automatic regulation that turns the stress responses on and turns them off. Robust stress responses allow ordinary people to endure the repeated and unpredictable demands of mundane daily life, as well as the extremes of war, without collapsing. We survive in part by flexibly raising and lowering our levels of physiological activity. Losing that nimble ability to adjust our stress responses can be lethal.[10]

The adaptive stress response begins in the hypothalamus, the coordinating center for basic drives. The first hormone in the stress response is corticotropin-releasing hormone (CRH), secreted from the paraventricular nucleus of the hypothalamus. When Gregory Hemingway heard his father say, "No? Well [your behavior] killed Mother," Greg experienced a burst of guilt, sorrow, and rage—his mind's reading of the burst of stress hormones that made his heart thump and his breathing tight and his head light under the image of himself as the agent of his mother's death. His father's words combined with Greg's thought, "I killed my mother?" to signal danger to his hypothalamus. Blood carries this squirt of CRH just a centimeter down to the pituitary gland. There the CRH tweaks the pituitary to secrete a second hormone, adrenocorticotropin hormone (ACTH).

ACTH then leaks into the bloodstream and out to all the organs, but only the adrenal glands sitting on top of the kidneys have the ACTH receptors that can read its potent message. Within seconds, the adrenal gland secretes adrenalin, also called epinephrine, and norepinephrine. These two hormones kick our hearts into action, raising our heart rate, blood pressure, breathing rate, cardiac output, and general sense of excitement or dread. The adrenal gland also gives us a jolt of steroids, mostly in the form of cortisol, the workhorse stress hormone that gives us the lift and surge of strength (or the illusion of strength, which is often good enough) we need to fight or flee. This hormonal disaster-management system requires an intact hypothalamus, pituitary, and adrenal gland, often called the HPA axis. This HPA axis is designed for sustained arousal throughout a hunt, fight, or run. Its signal to the heart, like all hormones, travels by blood and arrives slower than the signal from the amygdala to the heart, which travels by nerve fibers.

So, when all works well, sensory or cortical brain signals to the hypothalamus trigger CRH, which triggers ACTH, which triggers norepinephrine and cortisol, which race to help our hearts and lungs and muscles meet the challenge. Nerve pathways, hormone chains, and finally organs boot up for action. Multiple messengers and multiple secretion sites allow for regulation and self-regulation and several loops for feedback (for example, cortisol normally inhibits the hypothalamus from secreting too much CRH).

But when all does not work well, as in depression, there are many ways for the system to slip out of tune or dysregulate. Depressed people pour out more CRH than normal, the hormonal equivalent of persistent loud shouts to the body to prepare for the worst. Even when housebound, Gloria felt fear each day, and the simplest tasks demanded great efforts. Her stress-response system could not turn itself off. CRH injections are noxious to animals and would make you and me depressed and anxious for hours. Every day Gloria was probably secreting too much CRH.

Depressed people who secrete too much CRH also have larger, more active adrenal glands, which erratically produce bursts of adrenalin, norepinephrine, and cortisol. Their moods shift suddenly and without warning. Heart rates go up and down. Blood pressure goes up and down. And the usual negative feedback loop to the hypothalamus, by which high cortisol levels reduce CRH secretion to normal, fails to work effectively.[11] So the high-arousal state persists in erratic patterns instead of simply turning itself off. High arousal means higher resting heart rates, poorer control of heart rate, and overreactive blood-pressure responses to stress. The usual automatic mechanisms for keeping the cardiovascular system in tune wear out.

This faulty, trigger-happy stress-response system, which can't shut itself off, puts the rest of the body through the wringer too, especially the cardiovascular, gastrointestinal, and respiratory systems. Also called autonomic dysregulation, this state sets up some of the conditions that favor the development of heart disease and accounts for some of the common physical problems of depression, such as chest pains, palpitations, fatigue, headaches, diarrhea, cramping.[12] Over the long run of chronic stress and depression, persistent activation of the HPA axis, with high cortisol levels, weakens the immune response, opening the way for chronic inflammation, one of the key processes in coronary artery disease.

In addition to raising cortisol levels, depression may weaken the immune response and promote inflammation by blunting the parasympathetic nervous system, which normally helps constrain the inflammation process. Excessive inflammation in the coronary arteries accelerates the progression of coronary disease—in the early stages by establishing plaque in the walls of the arteries, and later by facilitating the rupture of plaques that then cause heart attacks. But the relationship between depression and inflammation goes both ways. Inflammation is usually a depressing experience, as we're reminded every time we get an infection and feel "down." In the laboratory setting, artificial injection of inflammatory proteins and cells in healthy people reliably produces transient depressive symptoms and behaviors. The same effect happens in other mammals. Though there's much we don't yet know about how this relationship between depression and the immune system works in people with heart disease, it's clear that the relationship plays an important role in the development and the progression of coronary artery disease.[13]

Active Ingredients in the Brain Soup

The "chemical imbalance" that Gloria talked about refers to the now common notion that depression involves a change in the usual balance of chemicals in our brains. More precisely, this notion implies a set of neurotransmitters that pass the electrical signals from one nerve to another in our brains. The neurotransmitters that carry the messages important to depression include, at the least, serotonin, norepinephrine, dopamine, acetylcholine, and glutamate. There are certainly others in this brain soup that we don't yet know about.

We know the most about serotonin and norepinephrine. In various ways each of these neurotransmitters also plays a role in the regulation of the cardiovascular system. For example, norepinephrine within the brain plays a major role in the regulation of depressed mood and anxiety; and norepinephrine outside the brain regulates blood pressure and heart rate. Serotonin, so important in the limbic system for mood regulation, also plays a crucial role in the bloodstream by controlling how readily platelets form blood clots, a key process in heart attacks.[14]

But depression messes with the usual recipe of brain neurotransmitters. Depression sours the soup by changing the mix of neurotransmitters in key parts of the brain and the rate at which they are produced and the number of receptors that can receive their signals. We now know how stress can switch genes on and off, disrupting the brain cells' production of the neurotransmitters, receptors, and enzymes that keep the system in balance. When serotonin activity falls below a critical threshold, not only does a person's mood drop but her platelets become sticky, sometimes sticky enough to add to the subtle process of forming tiny blood clots around the diseased parts of her arteries. We're beginning to learn about what's happening during depressive episodes to the genes that regulate serotonin activity.[15]

But the effort to explain depression on the basis of neurotransmitters has given us only partial answers. Our understanding of neurotransmitters has taught us that some classes of medications relieve depression better than others, and it has guided the development of new antidepressant drugs, to the great pleasure not only of many formerly depressed patients, but also of a few tycoons in the booming pharmaceutical industry. However, forty years of research on neurotransmitters in depression has not given us a comprehensive way of explaining what causes depression. For that explanation we'll need to look more on a scale that is both larger than the nerve synapse, such as Mayberg's model of limbic-cortical dysregulation, and smaller than the synapse, that is, within the nerve cells at intracellular messengers, altered DNA expressions, and new protein synthesis.

In 1997 Ronald Duman, professor of psychiatry and pharmacology at

Yale, proposed "a molecular and cellular theory of depression." This theory was based on observations in humans and animals that stress and depression slow down the synthesis of the proteins that keep hippocampal nerve cells remodeling themselves. The slow-down probably happened through low-grade or erratic elevations of cortisol, which inhibits neurogenesis in the hippocampus. This is the mechanism for the observed shrinkage or atrophy of the hippocampus in severely depressed patients by as much as 20 percent in some reports. Aging and opiate drugs also slow down neurogenesis. The longer the depression lasts, the greater the hippocampal atrophy.[16]

What does that shrinkage mean for you and me when we're depressed? It means that our memories fail us more often, usually our short-term memories, such as forgetting what you just told me you wanted for your birthday. And it means my embarrassment over this lapse is likely to be excessive. Our feelings shift more rapidly without apparent cause. We have to work harder to concentrate and harder to contain what feels like unreasonable emotional responses to benign situations. For an afternoon or a day or two, this level of effort may register as no more than a series of hassles. But after weeks and weeks of emotional and cognitive stumbling, the cycle takes on a life of its own, and that rut we call depression.

On the other hand, antidepressants, electroconvulsive therapy, and lithium increase the synthesis of BDNF and other neurotrophic factors in the hippocampus and prevent further atrophy, under some conditions helping the hippocampus regain its previous size and function. Learning, psychotherapy, and exercise also promote neurogenesis in the hippocampus. In animals the injection of BDNF into the brain reduces learned helplessness behavior. So, in addition to increasing neurotransmission across the synapse for more effective signal conduction from one nerve to the next, antidepressant treatments also foster protein synthesis that helps regenerate lost nerve connections in the hippocampus. This rewiring helps reregulate the limbic system's connections to the cortex.

Unlike the rapid process of increasing neurotransmission, which can happen within hours of taking an antidepressant, changing the rate of protein synthesis takes weeks. Most people who respond well to antidepressants notice a little improvement within a week or so, but the full benefit arrives three to four weeks after starting the therapeutic dose, about the time it would take for new protein synthesis to show its full effects. The same timing applies to the effects of psychotherapy and a sustained exercise regimen. The big benefit hits after three to four weeks of intensive treatment. That's when the cloud lifts and we begin to feel we have a fresh mind and a new brain, which in one small sense is literally true. Following the formation of new neural connections, the limbic and cortical pathways must then reorchestrate the balance that has been out of whack for so long. New structures, new functions. No wonder recovery from depression often requires several months, not days, after starting treatment.

Recovering the Brain and Heart

The good news from the biology of depression is that effective treatment of depression, in the form of antidepressant medications or psychotherapy, also returns the limbic system, the HPA axis, and the autonomic nervous system to normal functioning. When Gloria recovered from her depression through a combination of psychotherapy, medications, and prayer, her heart disease also improved. An angiogram of her heart in 2001, ten years after her heart attack, showed that her coronary arteries were normal, but because of that old heart attack, her heart wasn't pumping at full strength. She takes one medication for her blood pressure, one for her high cholesterol, and one for her depression. For the past several years she's had no problems with chest pain. She's still working on losing weight and eating healthier food, but she feels free of that terrifying fear now, and her faith is stronger. Depression no longer runs her life. And she has managed her risks for heart disease.

This quick tour of the biology of depression describes disruptions on every level of organization of the central nervous system. They include metabolic shifts in at least five major brain structures, abnormal hormone levels and feedback in the HPA axis, dysregulation of five neurotransmitter systems, and altered gene regulation of protein synthesis for neurogenesis in the hippocampus. In spite of the many biological processes associated with depression, key cause-and-effect questions remain unanswered. We have not yet studied these processes over long enough periods of time in large enough numbers of people. Like heart disease, the range of variation in the course, severity, duration, and type of depression argue for depression's being a complex set of disorders with multiple biological, as well as psychological and social, pathways. Now that we know the major biological pathways that break down during what is sometimes still called a nervous breakdown, the next step will be to study these processes during the course of the illness (many episodes over many years) across a range of people. Soon we'll find biologically distinct types of depression, and we'll find more effective ways to guide the brain back to its less tormented way of serving our minds and hearts.

CHAPTER 6

The Heart Has a Brain

The wife of the owner of the motel in which Martin Luther King, Jr, was assassinated collapsed with a cerebral hemorrhage the day of the assassination and died the following day.

One week after a medical checkup had pronounced a stubbornly independent, unmarried man in his seventies in good health, he called his family together and, over their protests, distributed his belongings, saying, "I don't need them anymore." As the last item was disposed of, he dropped dead before his astonished relatives.

A seventy-one-year-old woman arrived by ambulance at the emergency room, accompanying her sixty-one-year-old sister, who was pronounced dead on arrival. The older sister collapsed at the instant of receiving the news of her sister's death, shortly thereafter developed ventricular fibrillation, and died.

A fifty-five-year-old man died when he met his eighty-eight-year-old father after a twenty-year separation; then the father dropped dead.

Around 1964, at the peak of his medical and academic career, the voraciously curious George Engel, MD, began scouring the obituary pages in Rochester, New York, where he lived, and wherever he traveled.[1] By then in his sixties and a leader in the field of psychosomatic medicine, Engel had taken a rare path to studying the interactions between the mind and the body. He trained in both internal medicine and psychoanalysis. The question that troubled him when he started clipping obituaries was whether people really do, as we so casually say, get "scared to death" or "die for joy." Can grief break your heart? Do such deaths truly happen, or are they the fabrications of folklore? For the next six years Engel collected clippings about people who died in unusual circumstances, and by the time he finished, he had gathered 170 reports of people who had died suddenly, soon after some identified type of psychological distress.

In taking on the question of whether emotions can lead to sudden death, Dr. Engel was sticking his neck out. Though the idea had been popular in the eighteenth and nineteenth centuries, skepticism and ridicule had buried the possibility that feelings could be fatal, as the scientific method and the cellular model of disease took over modern medicine. Statistical probabilities alone could explain as mere coincidences the rare deaths that occurred soon after stressful events. Cause of death was to be decided at autopsy, where emotions are particularly hard to find. The dominant opinion in medicine held that, even among the living, emotions were unmeasurable and irrelevant to all but a few diseases.

Engel argued persuasively against this narrow view of disease, and eventually his view fundamentally revised medical education.[2] At the time, however, his imaginative and observant mind was fascinated by the unfashionable possibility that these rare and dramatic deaths, if they occurred at all, represented psychophysiologic accidents or extremes of normal functioning. He was peering at the normal by studying the extraordinary.

In his 1971 report on this project, Engel wrote that the stressful circumstances preceding the 170 deaths fell into three broad categories: loss of a close person, personal danger, and "happy endings" of reunion or triumph. The common denominator among those who died was an extreme feeling of overwhelming excitation combined with a sense of helplessness. Physicians attributed most of these deaths to sudden heart problems, either heart attacks or arrhythmias involving rapid acceleration or extreme slowing of heart rate. Often these people had existing heart disease, but sudden death also occurred in people with no apparent heart disease.

How could the mind do such a thing to the normal heart? In 1971 Engel made some educated guesses and called for more rigorous research. Since then, research has described the phenomenon of sudden cardiac death more precisely and identified several mechanisms. We know, for example, that sudden death in healthy adults following intense emotional experiences is exceedingly rare and impossible to predict, in light of how many intense emotional experiences we all endure without illness or death.

Our hearts are remarkably resilient, but they do register distress. Physicians in Israel's and Croatia's war zones have reported transient rises in the frequency of heart attacks among civilians following bombing raids, presumably linked to the immediate rise in the threat of death. Within six weeks, however, the heart attack rates returned to normal, suggesting rapid adjustment to persistent war stress by the people in these communities.[3]

Cardiologists have described a rare syndrome called "acute stress cardiomyopathy," which masquerades as a heart attack after intense emotional stress, except the heart muscle doesn't die. It is only "stunned" for a few days and recovers rapidly. The mechanism for this syndrome is similar to the mechanism for the rare tumor that killed Greg Hemingway's mother (see Chapter 4), namely the hormonal product of overwhelming excitation: toxic levels of adrenalin, which impair the ability of the heart muscle to contract.[4]

The Heart-Brain Connection

These rare and lethal events remind us of the close anatomical and physiological ties between the heart and the brain, between the cardiovascular and the central nervous systems. The body has a head and the heart has a brain. In fact, the cardiovascular system is so laced with nerves and the central nervous system is so laced with vessels that the boundary between the two cannot be precisely drawn. Platelets that regulate clotting contain neurotransmitters, such as serotonin, that regulate the platelets' behavior, making these platelets, in one sense, circulating pieces of the central nervous system. To nature, it's all one system. But we who need words to make sense of life break our biology into its apparent parts so we can talk about how the system works.

The conversation between the brain and the heart never ceases. Though the cardiovascular system also responds every second of every minute to shifts in the respiratory system and the endocrine system, the central nervous system wields the most sophisticated influence over the regulation of the heart and its vessels. As we look in greater detail at the extent of this regulatory influence, it will become clearer how the dysregulated brain of chronic depression exacts a heavy demand on the heart.

We've seen examples of how the mind works on the heart in extreme situations, like war, that lead to sudden death or heart attacks, but how about in our mundane daily lives? To find out just how real these mental demands on the heart can be in ordinary life, researchers at Duke University recruited 132 patients with coronary disease to wear heart monitors for forty-eight hours while they recorded their activities and emotions at home and at work. The heart monitors recorded a continuous electrocardiogram (ECG) tracing that was later analyzed for episodes of ischemia, or insufficient oxygen and blood flow to the muscle wall of the heart. The patients were unaware of what the tracing recorded and could guess based only on their own symptoms if they were having ischemia. Three times per hour for two days they kept records of physical activity and five emotions: tension, sadness, frustration, happiness, and feeling in control. The results? High levels of negative emotions (tension, sadness, frustration) roughly doubled the chance of having a transient ischemic episode within the next hour, similar in magnitude to the effect of moderate exercise. This is not to say that sadness or frustration will kill you—all these people did well during this short study. In fact, few of them were aware they were having ischemia, because it was brief, mild, and without symptoms. The ECG tracings in this study simply remind us that, in people with coronary disease, strong negative emotions transiently tax the ability of the heart to deliver enough oxygen to itself.[5]

It could be useful to know whether your heart slips into ischemia during mental stress. It doesn't happen to everyone or all the time, but for 40–70 percent of people with coronary disease, mental stressors provoke ischemia. Stressors that produce anger are particularly good triggers of ischemia. And the consequences can be dramatic. In one study that followed a group of 126 people with coronary disease, those who had laboratory evidence of mental stress-induced ischemia had almost three times the risk of developing a heart attack, needing bypass surgery, or dying by heart disease, compared to those who did not have ischemia under mental stress in the lab. This study and others have made the point that mental stress testing, like exercise stress testing, could identify a group of people with coronary disease who are at increased risk of bad outcomes but who have no other way of knowing of this risk. It would be similar to testing for the effects of physical stress—the exercise stress test has been a routine diagnostic tool for decades—which identifies people with coronary disease who are at risk of bad outcomes. But testing for mental stress–induced ischemia is currently available only in research settings and is not covered by health insurance.[6]

When I was in medical school during the late 1970s, we learned to view the cardiovascular system as the most sophisticated self-regulating system of elastic plumbing ever invented. This useful simplification underlies the common conception of hardening of the arteries as a problem similar to corrosion in the pipes under your sink. The thinking then was that heart attacks occurred when the sludge (cholesterol) in your blood narrowed your coronary arteries so much that red blood cells carrying oxygen couldn't pass through to the heart muscle on the other side of the narrowing. This focus on the mechanical difficulties in coronary disease led to powerful new surgical treatments like angioplasty that removed or reduced the blockage in the coronary artery. Maybe that would be enough.

The Slow Burn of Atherosclerosis

Chick Haydock watched helplessly over one long year as his law firm splintered and finally broke up. At fifty-nine and going strong, he was not about to slide into early retirement, but he also was not excited about starting out on his own. His sleepless moments at night began to burn with the hot gas of indigestion. He wondered if this was resentment smoldering. There was nobody to blame and nothing to do but get on with it. And so he did.

Chick started his own practice and made it work, but the tightness in his chest stayed with him. His doctor found that his blood pressure was up and sent him to a high-profile cardiologist, who did an angiogram and found severe narrowing in several of his coronary arteries. The cardiologist sent him to one of the best cardiac surgeons in town, who performed a coronary artery bypass graft, and after the surgery Chick felt so good that he resumed his law practice and his smoking, both of which had been a habit for almost forty years. "I pushed it aside," he said. "I felt I was going to live forever. I got myself into shape, was good with rehab, and practicing law full-time." He and his wife went ahead with the cruise they'd planned, and for the next five years he didn't have to bother about his heart.

When the gas pains came back five years later, he had another angiogram that showed one of his coronary arteries blocked. So through a long catheter inserted in an artery in his groin, his cardiologist slipped a stent, an artificial sleeve, into the blocked coronary artery and opened it up for instant relief. Grateful for this miraculous procedure that spared him a second operation, Chick began the rehab process once again. By now he had quit smoking, but his blood pressure and LDL cholesterol were both high. Then he discovered he had diabetes. Then, just a few months after he received the stent, it closed down. He had to have another bypass operation. Soon it became clear that he had narrowing of the arteries in his shoulder, his legs, and probably in his brain. His memory began to fail. His moods began to shift. Frustration mounted as the losses piled up: cases, workload, social life, short-term memories.

Chick Haydock's story is a common one. The mechanical problems get the quick fix by good plumbers, but that doesn't stop the slow burn of atherosclerosis. The mechanical model accounts for only a part of the disease process. To understand what happens to people like Chick Haydock, we've had to change our views and add to the traditional model two previously underappreciated dimensions of heart disease: First, hypertension and atherosclerosis are also driven by imbalances in the autonomic nervous system, the part of the central nervous system that manages the relatively automatic regulation of our internal organs (heart, lungs, digestive system, etc.); and second, atherosclerosis acts more like a disease of inflammation in the vessel walls than a plumbing problem. These dimensions of heart disease operate under the influence of biological links to depression.[7]

Anatomical Links between Heart and Brain

You can trace the anatomical links between the cardiovascular and the central nervous systems in Figure 6.1.[8] The heart and the brain, the dominant organs of each system, are served by branching systems of peripheral networks that match each other at every tributary of nerve and vessel. Dissect any mammal and you'll find that nerves follow vessels wherever they grow, in the developing embryo as well as in the healing wound of an adult. All our arteries are wired. The brain is always meddling in the affairs of the heart.

The heart itself has two nerve centers—concentrations of nerve tissue embedded in the muscle fibers—called the sinus node and the atrioventricular, or A-V, node. The automatic impulse that contracts the heart

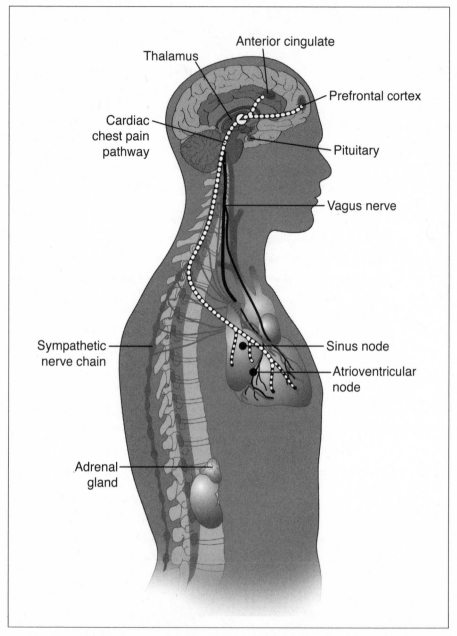

Figure 6.1. The Brain's Links to the Heart. Via the anatomical links between the cardiovascular and the central nervous systems, the brain is always meddling in the affairs of the heart.

with every beat begins high in the atrium at the sinus node, travels down through the A-V node, and then fans out through the ventricles below. This automatic heart rate is set to fire at a fixed rate, between fifty and ninety beats per minute. The actual heart rate, however, varies widely and sensitively in response to demands from the internal and external environment, and this adjusting is the work of nerves and hormones stimulating the sinus node. The brain is always meddling.

If the heart is the marionette of the brain, the vagus nerve is one of two main strings controlling the action. The vagus nerve connects the brainstem to the sinus node of the heart, passing along parasympathetic signals to slow down the heart rate. The more activity along the vagus nerve, the slower the heart rate, usually. The vagus nerve and the parasympathetic system put the brakes on the heart, usually gently, but on rare occasions, as Engel noted, so suddenly and extremely that the heart stops.

Clinical Tip 6.1: Take your autonomic nervous system for a walk. Though we can't reduce our blood pressure or heart rate by telling our sympathetic nerves to relax, we can change the balance of activity in our autonomic nervous systems in a number of ways. Moderate exercise, such as walking, particularly if done regularly, reduces the activity of our sympathetic nerves. Regular meditation also alters the balance of sympathetic and parasympathetic activity. And some medications, such as beta-blockers, benzodiazepines, and antidepressants, modify the tone of the autonomic nervous system. We can reduce the wear and tear on our cardiovascular system by learning to tone down our autonomic nervous systems with exercise, relaxation, meditation, and if necessary, medications.

The other main string controlling the action of the heart and balancing these parasympathetic signals is the web of sympathetic nerves to the heart from the upper half of a chain along the spinal cord. These sympathetic nerves play the accelerator role, charging the heart to speed up. Like the heart, all arterial vessels have this dual input, accelerator and brake. Arteries narrow or widen depending, in part, on the balance between sympathetic and parasympathetic tone in those nerves. Blood pressure reflects this balance. The sympathetic system transmits its signals for higher heart rates and narrower vessel diameters with the hormone and neurotransmitter norepinephrine, which also plays a major role in the limbic system of the brain and in depression. In contrast, the parasympathetic system transmits its signals for slower heart rates and vessel dilation with acetylcholine, also important in depression. Together the sympathetic and parasympathetic nerve networks are called the autonomic nervous system.

The brain keeps vigilant watch on what's happening down in the rest of the body. Most of this vigilance occurs beneath our awareness, literally, in brain structures that lie below our cortical centers of consciousness. As shown in Figure 6.1, the autonomic nervous system includes the sympathetic and parasympathetic divisions, plus the brain structures that regulate their activity. For example, fortunately, we can't sense modest rises in blood pressure or heart rate, can't hear heart murmurs, can't feel the more efficient pumping by the left ventricle while we're shoveling slush or running from the cops. We're spared awareness of our autonomic nervous system activity except when we're highly aroused or in danger. Like a fine automatic transmission, the autonomic nervous system manages the details for us. That's a good thing.

But, unfortunately, our lack of awareness sometimes goes too far, and the warning system fails. Though most people have chest pain that forces them to stop and rest and thus avoid a heart attack, heart attacks hit others, particularly women, without any chest pain at all, events often called "silent ischemia." Stuart Rosen and his colleagues at the Imperial College School of Medicine in London have described the pathways by which the brain registers cardiac sensations, such as ischemia and chest pain. In one study the brain areas that lit up with increased activity during chemically induced ischemic episodes were the thalamus, the hypothalamus, the prefrontal cortex, and the anterior cingulate cortex on the left—the same structures that regulate mood in depression.[9] Within the hypothalamus, the centers for cardiac chest-pain signals sit nested in the paraventricular nucleus, right next to the centers for the stress response that secrete CRH. Evolution had a good reason for pairing the stress-response system with the pathways for pain from the heart.

This pathway for chest pain—from the heart to the spinal cord to the thalamus, the hypothalamus, and the anterior cingulate—has been documented by other investigators. Note in Fig 6.1 that cardiac chest pain registers in the same general cortical areas as depression, the prefrontal cortex and the anterior cingulate, suggesting that our poetic tradition of linking grief of the soul with pain in the heart may have its roots in our neuroanatomy. These cortical areas are where we become aware of how our heart aches. The aching heart is more than a metaphor. "The anterior cingulate is the mapping site of cardiac pain, along with somatic and visceral pain," says Greg Fricchione, MD, associate professor of psychiatry at the Harvard Medical School. Depression happens to be mapped onto the same cortical areas as physical pain, suggesting an anatomic explanation for why pain is depressing, particularly chronic pain. Closing the loop back down to the heart, the anterior cingulate area is also directly connected by nerve tracts to the vagus nerve and to the sympathetic nerve chain.[10]

Rosen and his colleagues found evidence that the thalamus is the gatekeeper of chest pain signals, in charge of setting the threshold for communicating sensory information from the heart to the cortical centers for emotion and awareness. Normally the thalamus spares us from worrying about the adaptive fluctuations of the heart. But in silent ischemia the thalamus sets the threshold too high—the gate is rusted shut. The thalamus fails to alert the conscious mind to rest and seek help. This dangerous lack of information in the decision-making area of the brain often leads to infarction and death.[11]

There is also a group of people for whom the thalamic gating threshold for communicating cardiac pain signals to the cortex is set too low. Cardiologists have traditionally referred to this group as "Syndrome X," a term that confesses that the cause of their chest pain remains a mystery. These people report remarkable capacities to sense changes in their hearts that most people never sense (dye flowing in during angiograms, catheter tips tapping ventricle walls, balloon inflations during angiograms), and they report chest pain in the absence of any evidence of ischemia. Masters of the Ayurvedic tradition of eastern medicine may train a lifetime to achieve such exquisite sensitivity to their inner physical realms, but in our Western medical culture the consequences of such supersensitivity can prove more a curse than a blessing, earning those who seek help too often for these troubling sensations the label "hypochondriac."

However, Rosen's studies of brain scans of patients with Syndrome X suggest an anatomic explanation for the behavior of these patients. The overactive thalamus sends too many sensory signals to the cortex, which misreads them as chest pain, even though there's no ischemia. The thalamic gate has swung open too wide too often, and too many signals have leaked through to awareness.

The work of Rosen and his colleagues demands what Dr. Fricchione calls "a powerful paradigm shift." We now have to think of the brain as capable of wide variations in how it filters signals from the autonomic nervous system. Anxiety and depression usually magnify our perceptions of pain. Physical pain in general and chest pain in particular are common triggers for people with depression to seek help from emergency rooms and primary care doctors. During the months after a heart attack, depressed people report more chest pain than do nondepressed people.[12] Depression may alter the processing of pain signals at the level of the thalamus in a way that is similar to what Rosen observed in patients with Syndrome X. As the depression resolves, the heightened awareness of pain usually resolves too.

The New View of Atherosclerosis

In the traditional view, atherosclerosis, or hardening of the arteries, began with excessive levels of cholesterol circulating in the bloodstream and collecting on the arterial vessel walls. This collection of cholesterol bulges into the vessel, creating turbulence in blood flow at that narrowed site, as well as more deposits of cholesterol and eventually of calcium, forming a plaque that hardens and damages the wall of the artery. Circulating platelets eventually attack the plaque, triggering the formation of clots, which then clog the vessel either at the site of the plaque or downstream, resulting in a heart attack or stroke.

This model attributed the events of heart attacks and strokes to blockages in normal blood flow, but it left some key questions unanswered. Why do plaques form in some places more often than others? Why do small plaques contribute to heart attacks and strokes as much as large ones do? Why do heart attacks strike some people with low cholesterol?

The answers to these questions come from the recent shift in thinking about atherosclerosis as an inflammatory process rather than purely a plumbing problem.[13] The plaque behaves more like a sore than a dumping site. This means that the plaque functions as an injury functions, recruiting inflammatory cells and immune molecules to surround the site where low-density lipoprotein (LDL) particles, or "bad" cholesterol, leak into the artery wall. Under benign and transient conditions, the immune system cleans up these cholesterol deposits and the inflammation fades away with no lasting effects.

But when the conditions favoring atherosclerosis persist, the process accelerates unnoticed, often in many branches of the cardiovascular tree, such as the heart and the brain. Figure 6.2 shows how this accelerated process develops over many years.[14] It begins with excess LDL cholesterol circulating in the blood and diffusing through to the space between the endothelial cells and the muscle layer of the artery wall. This seepage happens more often near the branching forks in the arterial tree, where turbulent blood flow may shear the endothelial lining. These endothelial cells drag inflammatory cells and molecules from the blood to digest the LDL, forming "foam cells" filled with fat, the beginnings of the plaque. When conditions favorable for forming plaques persist for many months to years (high LDL cholesterol, high blood pressure, high levels of norepinephrine, elevated levels of inflammatory cells and molecules, activated platelets collecting along

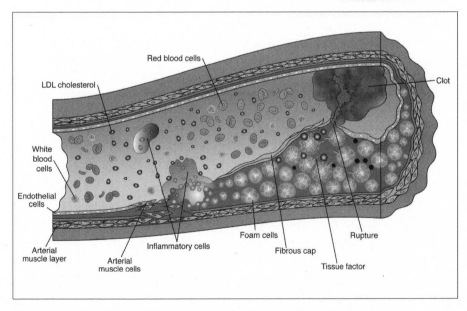

Figure 6.2. The Birth and Progression of a Plaque. A gradual tightening of plaque around the artery (shown here progressing from left to right) precedes the plaque rupture that causes most heart attacks.

the plaque), the foam cells accumulate and the plaque grows a fibrous cap. The plaque bulges both outward into the muscle layer of the artery and, after decades, inward into the lumen of the vessel, causing narrowing, more turbulence, and finally ischemia by constriction.

But most heart attacks don't occur at the end of this slow scenario of a gradual tightening of the plaque around an artery. Most heart attacks occur when an apparently benign or relatively small plaque suddenly cracks or breaks off. Clots form at the site of rupture or on the part that broke off. In an instant, a benign lesion becomes a dangerous one. This explains how people in their forties who were free of symptoms and unaware that they had heart disease, like Ted O'Reilly in Chapter 2 and Paula Volk in Chapter 1, could suddenly slump to the floor with a heart attack.

Smoking, obesity, and diabetes each adds to the inflammatory properties of LDL cholesterol, making it more likely to attract "foam cells" and add to plaque formation. High-density lipoprotein (HDL), or "good" cholesterol, on the other hand, helps carry away LDL and reduces the inflammatory properties of LDL. Your HDL, if you have enough of it, can protect you from your LDL.

Vascular Inflammation and Depression

This view of atherosclerosis means that during the years when plaques are developing in our arterial walls, we are often cooking a chronic, low-grade inflammation in many of the arteries throughout our bodies. In fact, as the level of vascular inflammation rises, the risk for heart attack or stroke rises. The best measure of vascular inflammation is a protein called C-reactive protein, or CRP. This marker of inflammation is a leading candidate to become the measure of the next major risk factor for coronary disease. In combination with cholesterol levels, CRP provides a potent predictor of heart disease. For example, whereas the highest CRP by itself increases cardiac risk 2.2 times higher than normal, and the highest LDL cholesterol by itself multiplies cardiac risk by about four, the highest CRP plus the highest LDL cholesterol readings raise a person's cardiac risk ninefold. That's a powerful effect. But we still don't know whether reducing inflammation and lowering CRP alone reduces this cardiac risk, because currently no medication or treatment specifically lowers CRP alone.[15]

Recent studies have begun to report how depression interferes with the normal immune response and promotes inflammation. For example, in one study men with a history of depression had more than two and a half times the chance of having an elevated CRP, compared to those with no depression history. Depression promotes low-grade inflammation by interfering with the regulation of the inflammatory process. Other reports have found that depression impairs the activity of some immune cells and key proteins in the inflammatory process, but the clinical importance of these changes has not been worked out. However, this effect of depression on many phases of inflammation represents another way in which depression can fuel the atherosclerotic process anywhere in the cardiovascular tree. In one large study, high CRP alone did not predict a later heart attack, but depressed mood combined with high CRP nearly tripled the risk for later heart attack.[16]

Clinical Tip 6.2: Insist on comprehensive treatment of heart disease. Because depression may make heart disease harder to treat, you should know what amounts to good or comprehensive treatment of heart disease, and insist with your doctor on trying for nothing less. Appendix H offers a brief guide to Web resources on current treatments for heart disease, and references for further reading.

Sympathetic Overactivity

Stevo Julius, MD, ScD, is a ruddy, energetic man in his seventies with unruly grey hair, a fuzzy beard, the faintest remnant of a central European accent, and an endearing impatience with the traditional thinking of his colleagues. Almost forty years ago after obtaining his two doctoral degrees in Zagreb, Yugoslavia, he came to the University of Michigan, where he has built a prolific research and clinical career focused on hypertension, particularly the role of the nervous system in hypertension. For twenty-five years he was chief of the Division of Hypertension in the Department of Internal Medicine at the university. In his honor the International Society of Hypertension has established the Stevo Julius Award for Excellence in Hypertension Education.

In spite of his considerable influence in his field, Dr. Julius remains baffled and amused by colleagues who don't listen to him, the ones who pay too little attention to the heart rates of their patients. "It's cheap, it's easy," he says. "You just take the pulse. Resting heart rate is a good measure of autonomic imbalance. But the idea has not caught on." The idea he refers to is the practice of assessing the hypertensive patient's autonomic nervous system. Most doctors make sure the heart rate isn't over one hundred or under fifty, but within that range they waste little time interpreting heart rates. That is partly because heart rates vary widely by person and setting and time. But most doctors also don't think of the heart rate in this range as an indicator of what the autonomic nervous system is doing. Julius thinks that's a mistake when caring for patients with heart disease:

> In clinical practice, the presence of tachycardia [high heart rate] is often viewed as a sign of benign "nervousness." . . . To the contrary, tachycardia is a strong predictor of excessive coronary morbidity and of cardiovascular mortality.[17]

What is your heart rate right now while you are at rest? Mine at the moment is sixty-four beats per minute. I don't have hypertension, but if I did, that heart rate would add nothing to my risk for heart disease. However, a condition that increases my resting heart rate to seventy-five beats per minute would put me in the second-highest category of risk for heart disease, and increasing it to eighty-five puts me in the highest category, more than doubling my risk, independent of any other risk factors. Just as a high idle speed is bad for my car engine, it really matters how fast my heart is racing when I'm resting. A difference of ten or twenty beats per minute, if sustained over the years, could change my life.

Increased resting heart rate is associated with high blood pressure, high blood glucose, high blood lipids, and obesity, which are all major risk factors for atherosclerosis.[18] Dr. Julius and his colleagues trace the high heart rate to the sympathetic nervous system, that chain of nerves along the thoracic spine that automatically jumpstarts the mechanisms for high alert. When the sympathetic nervous system is overactive and the parasympathetic system is underactive, as often happens in depression, one of the results is a high resting heart rate.

Another result is the gradual development of high blood pressure. The same signals that makes the heart beat faster make the arterial walls contract to raise the pressure, namely higher levels of norepinephrine or faster firing in the sympathetic nerves to the heart and the arteries. Even mild elevations of resting heart rate predict the later development of high blood pressure.

Several other consequences of sympathetic overactivity for sustained periods (months to years) lay the groundwork for the acceleration of atherosclerosis. The heart wall thickens, particularly around the left ventricle, which does most of the pumping. Think of this effect as nature's attempt to bulk up the heart to pump against the greater resistance of higher blood pressure. This is not a good thing, in general, because more muscle requires more oxygen, which is already in scarce supply for people with coronary disease, and thicker heart walls are more prone to heart attacks, arrhythmias, and sudden death. This bulking effect also occurs throughout the whole cardiovascular tree, adding to the hardening of the arteries. The whole system becomes less elastic or less "compliant" when the sympathetic tone is too high.[19]

And the blood thickens. The number of red blood cells rises after prolonged sympathetic overactivity. The best guess is that this thickening of the blood results from the greater leakage of fluid out of the vessels at the level of the capillaries, partly under greater blood pressure and partly because increased sympathetic tone makes capillaries more leaky. This rise in red blood cell numbers adds to the tendency to form clots, not what you want on top of atherosclerosis.

Increased heart rate means increased injury to arterial walls. The more rapid shifts in blood flow result in more frequent wear and tear on the lining of coronary arteries. Stress hormones change the way the endothelial lining cells work and make the lining leaky, opening the cells to injury. Injured endothelial cells become sites for repair and inflammation, potentially seeding the growth of atherosclerotic plaques. Plaques tend to form at these sites of turbulent fluid dynamics, and turbulence flips the caps off plaques, even young plaques, leading to blockages and sudden heart attacks.[20] But if you lower your heart rate over many months through exercise or medications, you can reduce the number and severity of these plaques. A lower heart rate means lower risk of cardiovascular death.[21]

Paradoxically, sympathetic overactivity may foster obesity.

At first glance, cranking up the engine, the way sympathetic activity cranks up the heart, should burn up the calories and reduce the likelihood of weight gain. But several studies have observed the opposite, namely that high heart rate and high blood pressure precede weight gain, suggesting that the first problem may have been sympathetic overactivity, which later led to the weight gain. High levels of cortisol, which often accompany chronic stress, foster the paunch or the beer belly, a different distribution of fat than usual, and one particularly common in people with heart disease. The other common scenario occurs when obesity leads to increased sympathetic activity and high blood pressure.[22]

So sympathetic overactivity, one feature of the biology of depression, contributes to heart disease by raising heart rate, raising blood pressure, beefing up the walls of the heart and arteries, thickening the blood with red blood cells, injuring the walls of the coronary arteries, and fostering obesity. Long before coronary disease declares itself a problem to the patient or the doctor, two important conditions for atherosclerosis persist off and on for many years: sympathetic overactivity and chronic low-grade inflammation. And depression contributes to both of these.

CHAPTER 7

The Vicious Cycle: Behavioral and Biological Links

I'd been seeing Bea Hock at the Wyoming family Practice Clinic about once a month for nine months when one day last May, by chance, I saw something about her that I should have seen from the start. On that day she happened to be one of six people on my schedule, and the third depressed, overweight, middle-aged woman. At the end of the day when I looked closer at the problem lists of these three women, I saw that, in addition to depression, each one had at least two of the following other major cardiac risk factors: smoking, diabetes, high cholesterol, high blood pressure, or nearly no physical activity. Even if you're looking for it, as I thought I had been, it's easy for mental health clinicians to miss cardiac risk factors in people who haven't had full-blown heart attacks and don't yet wear the "I have heart disease" sign on their charts. Bea Hock had never shown me any concern about heart disease, nor had her family physician called it to my attention, aside from brief notes on her blood pressure and cholesterol.

When I visited Ms. Hock at her two-bedroom ranch-style home where she lives alone in a suburb near the clinic, her impeccable house showed no sign of her six-year-old granddaughter, who had spent the morning there. Bea Hock sat me down at her round table and brought out a couple of family pictures. She told me that growing up she felt "set apart" from her three siblings, the only one of the four kids who got their mother's blues streak. Her mother was an ardently Catholic woman who believed that "suffering is a way of life," there is a devil, and God will punish you. After years of debilitating depression, her mother took her life by overdose at sixty-one, stunning the family, including seventeen-year-old Bea, who felt she was the only person in the family who had understood her mother's melancholic misery.

At family parties and celebrations, Bea never understood or felt the excitement she saw in other people. "I just didn't get it," she says now. Bea was "the gloomy one" and, ever since second grade, the fat one. Over the last twenty years, Bea's own depression, in recent years riddled by panic attacks, finally disabled her at age forty-seven after an effective career in financial management. Only her vow to spare her own two daughters the legacy of a mother's suicide has kept her from following her mother's example.

Bea Hock is a survivor, one of many private heroes of the undeclared war on depression. She has participated in psychiatric treatment in several settings for more than ten years, but every appointment with me over the past two years at the clinic has been packed with tears and laughter. Now at fifty-seven she's sixty pounds overweight, still struggling to keep depression at bay, and at times terrified by life outside her house. She's battle weary, but she never misses a chance to laugh at her troubles. Somewhere along the way she picked up a touch of her father's humor.

Clinical Tip 7.1: Don't let depression interfere with preventing heart disease. Technically, Ms. Hock does not yet have heart disease. She has no symptoms and her only angiogram, seven years ago, was normal. But she has plenty of risk factors: a family history of an early heart attack, overweight, physical inactivity, high blood pressure, high cholesterol, and chronic stress. She's in a position to prevent heart disease by improving any of the last five of them. Recently, her focus on depression and her frustration with the partial effectiveness of depression treatments have distracted her and her doctors from more aggressively working to reduce her cardiac risk factors. Behavior change is tough but possible. During periods of depression, patients often need more help with the work of prevention. We don't have to wait for a life-threatening event to tap into the motivation to change these behaviors. Ms. Hock needs a comprehensive heart disease prevention plan and some attentive coaching.

Last week I asked her about the rings on each of her ring fingers. "These are my war medals," she said, holding them up and smiling, "one from my first husband, this other from my second, and these extra two stones in the first one are from the man I loved more than either of them, the one who was really good to me until he died of cancer and I went under. That's my luck with men." She laughed and I smiled.

Bea Hock's blood pressure's high, her cholesterol's high, her weight's high, and she hasn't broken a sweat from exercise in years. She remembers clearly her father's heart attack at age forty-four and his bypass operation at fifty-four. Every day Bea takes a pill for her blood pressure, a pill for her cholesterol, and three for her depression. She knows she's something of a time bomb, but she doesn't fret about heart disease much. For her, depression poses a more urgent daily threat. "I wouldn't care if I had a heart attack tomorrow," she said with a hint of a wink. "Just make it quick." For many people with depression and heart disease, the burden of depression undermines the inclination to prevent heart disease.

Models of Illness

Every day in primary care clinics across the country people like Ms. Hock, men and women in their forties and fifties, come for help with a similar cluster of problems: high blood pressure, too much weight, too little exercise, high cholesterol, sometimes diabetes or smoking—often associated with impressive amounts of anxiety or depression. This clustering of psychological and physical problems is more than an occasional coincidence. It is heart disease waiting to happen. These problems share multiple biological pathways. One common combination of these problems, recently labeled the "metabolic syndrome," is linked to both distress and coronary disease.[1]

We can now pull together into a coherent working model the behavioral and biological links between depression, stress, and coronary heart disease. These linking pathways provide a framework for assessing risks for heart disease and risks for depression, and they suggest starting points for designing treatments. Whether we're patients, doctors, or research pharmacologists, the mechanisms of illness can suggest treatment strategies. The better we understand how depression, stress, and heart disease affect each other, the more likely we are to find ways to break the cycle.

But first a cautionary word about models of illness. Science loves models. It can't do without them. Models are creative oversimplifications that set up the questions to be tested. But we cannot reduce the biopsychosocial dimensions of chronic illnesses to phrases, boxes, and arrows without losing some of the truth. However, the working model of depression and heart disease presented here makes the point that, within the complex tangle of factors linking these two disorders, it is now possible to trace a few plausible pathways that make intuitive sense, are supported by the evidence, lend themselves to scientific study, and can guide the planning of treatment. We now have a road map.[2]

As we move through this series of figures, it helps to keep in mind a few assumptions. First, the lists of risk factors in these figures suggest possibilities, and the combinations of factors that actively contribute to the development of heart disease vary from person to person and from time to time. These lists provide selected examples, a kind of shorthand for the larger number of possibilities in any group of factors that contribute to the link between depression and heart disease.

Second, the relative importance of any single factor will vary over time. Smoking half a pack a day for a few years in your twenties may be cool for your social life without harming your heart to any great extent, but if you're still smoking in your forties when a back injury forces you to abandon your job as a tree surgeon, smoking half a pack a day may suddenly accelerate the development of heart disease. Now that you're inactive and in pain and stressed about losing your job, smoking becomes more toxic to your heart than it would have been in your twenties, or if you hadn't been injured.

Third, cause-and-effect relationships between two factors may shift over the course of the development of heart disease. For example, physical inactivity may initially lead to obesity, which then further restricts physical activity in an escalating fashion. Here's the vicious cycle at work. If depression turns me into a sloth, the fatness that follows will be depressing, and around we go. These figures read from left to right with the implication that time also moves in that direction, but a number of late-developing factors also influence factors that may have initially preceded them. We'll see in Chapter 8 how the process looks when it moves in reverse, from right to left, when heart disease triggers depression. But first, the earlier part of the cycle.

Four Levels of Effects

The point in Figure 7.1 is that depression can exacerbate heart disease on four possible levels, depending on the stage of the illness: In the early stages, (A) depression may contribute to high-risk behaviors, such as smoking or overeating, and (B) depression may directly alter the biological aspects of cardiovascular functioning, such as by raising resting heart rate. Later, (C) depression may exacerbate already existing early forms of other diseases that contribute to heart disease, such as diabetes or hypertension. And (D) depression may aggravate heart disease after it has developed.[3] These possibilities underlie the organization of the model presented in Figures 7.2–7.4, with psychological factors working through behavioral and biological factors to set up early disease conditions that promote the development of atherosclerotic heart disease, such as coronary disease, congestive heart failure, and stroke.

In Figure 7.2, some of the major and minor cardiac risk factors dis-

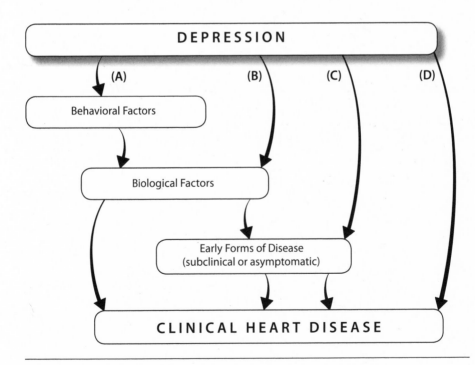

Figure 7.1. Four Levels of Depression's Effects on Heart Disease

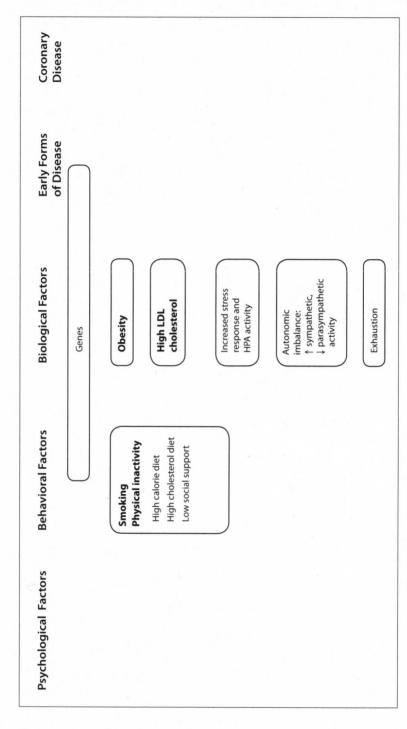

Figure 7.2. Early Risk Factors in Coronary Disease

cussed in Chapters 2 and 6 are grouped into sets of behavioral and biological factors. (The established major risk factors for coronary disease discussed in Chapter 2 and 3 are identified by bold type in Figures 7.2–7.4.)
In addition to the two major behavioral risk factors for coronary disease,
smoking and physical inactivity, poorly controlled diets and social withdrawal because of depression add to the behavioral burden. Though she
never smoked, Beatrice Hock ate more junk food when she was depressed.
She saw fewer friends, drifted away from her family, and spent more day-
time hours in bed.

Tied to these behaviors and at the top of the list of biological factors,
genes affect everything, though we don't yet know in detail how and we
can't name more than a few of the specific genes likely to affect both depression and heart disease. Major depression and coronary disease are both
familial diseases to which genes contribute substantially. Bea's father died
young of a heart attack and her mother died early from suicide. Some genes
direct the mechanics of cardiovascular functioning, and others promote or
protect us from risky behaviors. Genes related to serotonin play a role in
both depression and coronary disease. Because serotonin affects the vascular tone of vessels of the heart, and serotonin not only affects the tendency
of platelets to form blood clots but also regulates mood centers in the limbic system of the brain, recent research has zeroed in on the genes that control the serotonin transporter. Variations in the activity of this set of genes
may help us understand the biological bridge between depression and heart
disease.[4]

In turn, behaviors and stressful events can switch on the expression of
genes that contribute to heart disease. For example, poorly controlled diets
can reveal genetically inherited forms of obesity and hypercholesterolemia.
Stressful life events may combine with a genetic vulnerability for low serotonin transport activity to trigger clinical depression. The genetic regulation
of nicotine receptors may make smoking irresistible for some people. And
at the extreme end of the shyness spectrum, loners are more likely to lose
their precious few social supports when depressed, making recovery from
depression much tougher. And what if you're a shy, overweight smoker—
how many genes related to those factors are promoting the depression and
heart disease link? We don't know yet, but soon we'll be able to name at
least some of the specific genes that influence most of the important risk
factors for coronary disease, including depression.[5]

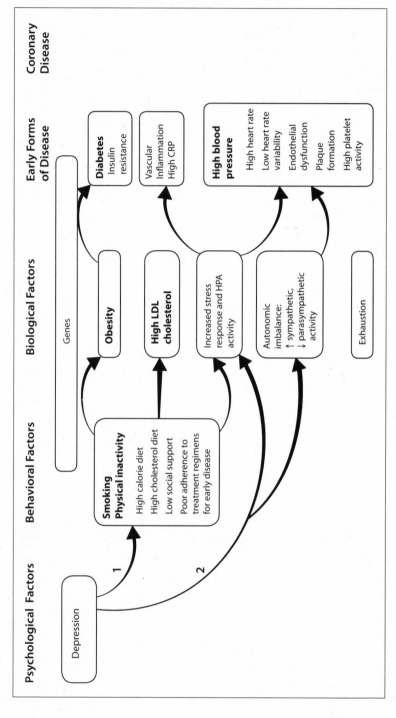

Figure 7.3. Two Pathways from Depression to Early Forms of Disease

Other biological factors in this bridge between depression and heart disease include disruptions of our stress hormones and of our autonomic nervous system. The increased stress-response hormones and HPA activity, such as the elevated cortisol so characteristic of severe depression, often lead to imbalances in the autonomic nervous system. In particular, sympathetic overactivity may contribute to higher blood pressure, higher resting heart rates, and exaggerated physiological responses to stress. And in several studies, chronic physical exhaustion, apart from the fatigue associated with depression, has predicted the development of coronary disease and death.[6] Bea's high blood pressure, her easy fatigability, and her low tolerance for stress all reflect an autonomic nervous system that is easily thrown out of balance. Instead of the regulation happening automatically, she has to exhert effort every day to stay in balance.

In Figure 7.3, we add depression to the picture and see two pathways by which depression can contribute to early forms of other diseases, conditions such as diabetes, vascular inflammation, and hypertension. The first pathway (1) operates through behavioral factors, which then lead to biological factors that favor the development of early forms of disease. We saw in Chapter 3 how depression exacerbates four of the six major risk factors for coronary disease, often through promoting high-risk behaviors. With early forms of disease now in the picture, we must add a new item to the behavioral factors: poor adherence to treatment regimens for diseases such as diabetes or hypertension and for conditions such as obesity and hypercholesterolemia. Sticking with any regimen is tough for many of us, but when the hopelessness or fatigue or memory impairment of depression reduces adherence to these treatment regimens, depression accelerates the development of heart disease.

The second pathway (2), the neuroendocrine pathway, more directly reflects the biological changes inherent in major depression. If these biological disruptions persist long enough (and we don't yet know how long that is), then the conditions that favor the development of coronary disease begin to develop, such as a rise in the heart rate, a drop in the heart-rate variability, prolonged endothelial dysfunction and plaque formation in the coronary arteries—all in a setting that promotes vascular inflammation and elevations of C-reactive protein (CRP). The presence of high blood pressure or diabetes fuels this process further.

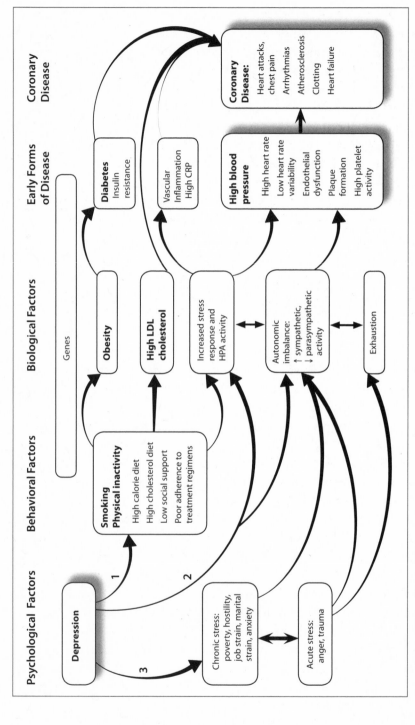

Figure 7.4. Plausible Pathways from Depression to Coronary Disease

In Figure 7.4, we see the emergence of clinical heart disease from early forms of disease, and a third pathway linking depression to various forms of chronic stress and anxiety. This model makes several points. First, coronary disease is the product of many factors, some close and some quite distant in time from when the first cardiac symptoms appear. The chest pain, heart attacks, arrhythmias, atherosclerosis, abnormal clotting, and heart failure that are characteristic of coronary disease are the measurable final products of a long series of silent or often unrecognized biological events, fostered in part by psychological and behavioral factors.[7] Because the relative importance of each factor and the sequence of events vary from person to person, effective treatment of heart disease for a particular person depends on knowing which factors have been or are currently in play.

Second, psychological factors such as depression work through many possible biological mechanisms, some more direct than others, to influence the development and progression of coronary disease: sympathetic overactivity, increased platelet activity, low heart-rate variability, increased inflammation. No single mechanism or pathway is likely to be important without some influence from the others, and no single treatment can be sufficient. So treatment must aim at many targets in the psychological, behavioral, and biological areas to shut down the disease process.

Third, this is a complex and dynamic set of systems. Studies of the relationship between depression and coronary disease, depicted on the left and right in Figure 7.4, must measure the many intervening psychosocial, behavioral, and biological factors which modify and mediate this relationship, and they must measure how the relative importance of these factors shifts over time. That's a tall order. Studies of complex relationships over long spans of time require large groups of research subjects and large coffers of funds. Fortunately, a handful of studies have begun collecting good data on these behavioral and biological risk factors for coronary disease in various samplings of the U.S. population. At this point the findings from these studies remain too spotty to answer the important questions about specific psychological and behavioral mechanisms linking depression and coronary disease, but answers will likely come in the next five to ten years.[8]

Fourth, an alternate pathway (3) in this model emphasizes depression's relationship to other psychosocial factors—the chronic and acute stresses of poverty, anger, marital strain, loneliness, morbid worries, and sleepless nights. The little tortures of our endless weeks add to the toll on our hearts. The real culprit may be prolonged distress of any kind, or a combination of distress and isolation, as in Denollet's type D personality, described in Chapter 2; for now, depression is simply one of the better defined and better studied forms of distress that aggravates heart disease.[9]

Clinical Tip 7.2: Identify the factors that have contributed to your current condition. Using a copy of Figure 7.4, circle each of the factors that have contributed to your current condition (or that of your family member or your patient). Take note of where the circles cluster and the factors for which you may need more information or treatment (see Figure 7.5). Clustering of circles around active factors in the left two columns suggests the need for psychological and behavioral interventions to prevent the development of coronary disease. Clustering of circles in the three columns on the right suggests the need for biological interventions to prevent the progression of early or existing coronary disease. Scattering of circles across the five columns points to the need for a comprehensive treatment plan that combines psychosocial and biological interventions. Figure 7.4 can also serve as a quick checklist for making sure that you're not overlooking the important factors that play a role in your heart disease. Do not assume that your doctor has checked on all these factors; review the list together.

Once coronary disease has appeared in the form of angina, heart attack, or an abnormal angiogram of the coronary arteries, the same mechanisms that set up atherosclerosis make it worse. In fact, the importance of these risk factors increases once clinical heart disease has declared itself, and their effects are now more measurable in terms of abnormal functioning or tissue damage. Persistent smoking, high cholesterol, and poorly controlled diabetes accelerate the coronary disease process, hastening the progression to angina, heart attacks, or death. Many of the standard treatment strategies for coronary disease are based on the assumption that the most effective way to manage coronary disease over the long run is to reduce the factors that contributed to its development.[10]

Reviewing the Pathways in Action

Figure 7.5 is my version of the pathways figure for Beatrice Hock, with my notes in the margins. Since I knew her well, it took me about two minutes to do this checklist, and it tells me a number of useful things that I had not realized about the treatment plan that her family doctor and I have developed for her, even though I've been working with both of them for more than a year. First, I knew she had chronic and relatively severe major depression that has been stable for the past year, but it's been a few months since I checked on the severity of her depressive symptoms. Stability is not the same as full remission of symptoms. I should check on severity at the next appointment and talk with her again about how we could try to reduce her symptoms further (bright-light therapy? a more effective antidepressant medication? more intensive psychotherapy?). We should never back off from the effort to reduce the depression symptom burden, especially in chronic depression complicated by high risks for heart disease.

Second, I need more information on how well Bea sticks to her cardiac regimen. I've never talked with her about her eating habits and how hard it has been to change them. We've talked about increasing her exercise by walking and she's making progress there, but is she on a low-salt diet for her hypertension and a low-calorie diet for her weight? And how consistently does she take her medications for hypertension and high cholesterol? I'd overlooked these things. And I may be able to help her improve her adherence to her cardiac regimen. We should at least try.

With Ms. Hock's strong family history of early heart disease, her weight of 223 pounds (she's only five feet three), her still borderline-high LDL cholesterol while on a cholesterol-lowering medication, and her borderline-high blood pressure on an antihypertensive medication, I know that these four biological factors continue to put her in the high-risk category for developing coronary disease. How long is the fuse on her "time bomb"? She hasn't been bothered by any symptoms of heart disease recently, but the picture would be more serious, more urgent, if she had a high fasting blood glucose indicating insulin resistance or early diabetes. If her CRP is high, indicating inflammation in her cardiac arteries, that would raise her risk even more. Why hadn't we checked these labs? My conclusion from this quick exercise is that we're not being aggressive enough in our efforts to change Ms. Hock's high-risk behaviors and her high-risk biology for her

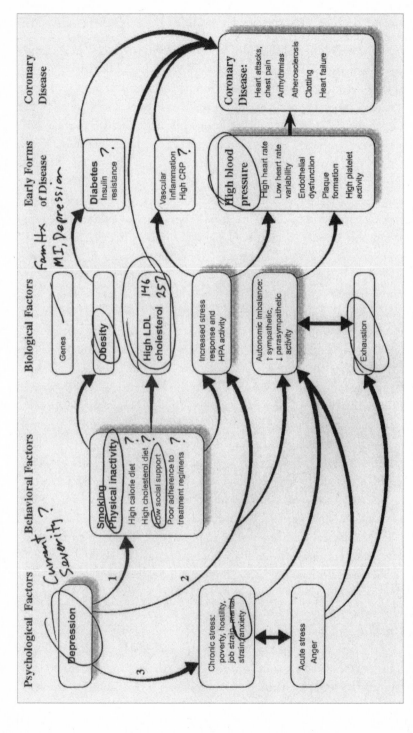

Figure 7.5. Active Pathways from Depression to Coronary Disease for Ms. BH, Age Fifty-seven

heart disease. We could be doing more, and we shouldn't wait for her to have chest pains or a heart attack to do more.[11]

These pathways give us a systematic way of thinking about the many steps from depression to heart disease. They show us a number of ways to break the links. And they chart the sequences that researchers must study to spell out in greater detail how these mechanisms work. Through the complexity of this understanding comes hope and the promise of better treatments. But before discussing treatments in detail, we must take stock of another level of complexity, for this interactive disease process often operates in reverse as a cycle of influences. If weight gain was once a consequence of Beatrice Hock's depression, it is now a contributing cause for her high blood pressure, which may contribute to depression by a new mechanism. In addition to reading the figures in this chapter from left to right, it helps to read them from right to left, as we will in Chapter 8.

CHAPTER 8

Is Heart Disease Depressing? The Vascular Depression Hypothesis

For most people, heart disease is not depressing. We are, for the most part, a remarkably resilient species, even when we face a lethal illness. Tom Geraci still can't imagine a bypass operation making him depressed. Norman Cousins, editor of the *Saturday Review* and later professor of medicine at UCLA, where he wrote *The Healing Heart* and *Head First: The Biology of Hope*, exemplified resilience in the face of heart disease, a threat which finally killed him but never depressed him. Most people with heart disease do not develop serious depressive disorders. However, for the sizable minority who do experience depression after developing heart disease—in the United States, some 600,000 people every year, or 40 percent of those who have heart attacks or severe angina, people like Paula Volk (Chapter 1) and Chick Haydock (Chapter 6)—the compelling questions are, How did this happen? And, What can we do about it?

Everybody seems to know somebody who has been laid low by heart disease in some dramatic fashion. One seventy-two-year-old man I spoke to, Harry Finian, told me, "Every person I've known who got heart disease—and I've known a lot—has had trouble with depression. Talk to my brother-in-law, my cousins, every one of them." Though Finian may be stretching the truth for effect, his observation is common. In general, people who stop to think about the link between depression and heart disease more readily acknowledge that heart disease could "cause" depression than that depression could "cause" heart disease. It makes intuitive sense that heart disease could be depressing, the way any life-threatening illness could rob us of hope.

But when I ask these same people, even my medical colleagues, how that connection might work, most either admit they have no idea or they fumble around with vague notions of the universal fear of death or loss of self-esteem from illness, explanations that don't have much to do specifically with heart disease or its biology. To many it remains a mystery how heart disease, more than most other chronic illnesses, could cause such sudden onsets of depression in people who were not bothered by depression in the first forty or fifty years of their lives.

Harry Finian had plenty of reason to expect that heart disease would kill him, but until his first chest pains hit, he never thought heart disease could get him down. With a Purple Heart from the Korean War, and as a father of five and a career salesman for a surgical supply company in Columbus, Ohio, Harry Finian had seen plenty of life and death by the time chest pains first hit him at sixty. But he had no personal experience with depression, and depression didn't run in his family the way heart disease did. Finian had watched his father die suddenly of a heart attack at sixty-five, his older brother die suddenly of a heart attack at fifty-six, and his younger brother survive a "six-way bypass operation" just a few years before. "Fourteen of my first cousins died of heart attacks—all men. None of the women," he said. That makes him, now surviving into his seventies, feel like the lucky one.

Though he'd smoked a pack a day for forty years—"the army got me started with free cigarettes in Korea"—and he knew his family history of heart disease all too well, he was still surprised when the cardiologist who evaluated his chest pains told him he needed an angioplasty right then to open a blockage in his coronary artery. He hadn't been aware of any problems with his blood pressure or his cholesterol, and he'd figured that as long has he had no symptoms, he had nothing to worry about. The cardiologist performed the angioplasty and it helped, but just a few months later the chest pains came back, and the cardiologist repeated the angioplasty to open up the same blockage at the same site. Chest pains came back again, and finally the next year Finian had a bypass operation. That fixed the problem.

But in the meantime his life had changed. Within weeks of the first angioplasty, Harry's normally athletic level of energy dropped and with it his mood. "The first is shock, next is fear, then the depression sets in," he said. "It was despair, and uncertainty—I asked lots of questions of my first cardiologist and got few answers. I lost my enthusiasm for work and fun. I just didn't care anymore. I stopped doing everything."

Harry struggled to recover on his own, thinking this was just what heart disease did to people. Finally, after his bypass operation relieved his chest pains but not his depression, he went to see a psychiatrist chosen by his family doctor. Harry didn't like the psychiatrist; she seemed more interested in giving him lots of drugs than helping him with his despair. So he quit after the second appointment, figuring he'd have to recover from the depression on his own. It took him most of the next year to regain his earlier level of activity at work and to recover from the worst of the depression, but some of the fatigue lingered and he never regained his enthusiasm for work. Now, at seventy-two, he's enjoying retirement on nine medications for his heart disease.

Vascular Depression

Was Harry Finian's depression anything more than a coincidence or the common tough time anyone might go through when coping with a potentially lethal diagnosis? In retrospect it is likely that he developed what is now being called vascular depression, a possibility his doctors did not investigate because at the time there was no clinical term for this condition. The term surfaced in the late 1990s as a potential new subtype for depression. A geriatric psychiatrist, George Alexopoulos, and his colleagues at Cornell University first articulated the hypothesis that depression could be caused by cerebrovascular disease, or hardening of the arteries in the brain.[1] They noted the high rates of depression in elderly people with hypertension, coronary disease, or vascular dementia. They proposed that decreased blood flow to the areas of the brain responsible for mood regulation could be the mechanism that explains the high rates of depression among people with cerebrovascular disease.

Though depression frequently develops after strokes, several recent studies have also found an alarmingly high rate of "silent strokes" in elderly depressed populations, in the range of 80–90 percent. Silent strokes reflect loss of blood flow to tiny areas of the brain, small infarcts that do not result in obvious physical impairments. Imagine a Swiss cheese pattern of tiny bubbles scattered here and there around the brain where before there had been healthy brain cells. In general, elderly people with depression show more evidence of this "silent" diffuse vascular disease in the brain than do elderly people without depression.

The location and pattern of these tiny bubbles determines what kinds of effects they cause, if any. When these patterns of ischemia affect the anatomic circuits that regulate depression, from the deepest areas of the limbic system, such as the hypothalamus and hippocampus, to the prefrontal and cingulate areas of the cortex, the ischemia causes changes in serotonin and norepinephrine transmission in these areas that are similar to the changes seen in animal models of depression. As with the more common forms of depression that start earlier in life, brain-imaging studies have recently begun to describe the anatomical and physiological patterns of overactivity and underactivity associated with late-onset major depression and vascular depression.[2]

For the patient and the clinician, vascular depression boils down to two key features: evidence of vascular disease, whether in the heart, the brain, or the peripheral vessels (as in hypertension); and late-onset (after fifty) depression, or a change in the course of depression in people who had early-onset depression. In several ways vascular depression differs from the more common type of major depression, which starts in the teens or twenties (hence the label "early onset") and which affects women more often than men. In contrast, vascular depression starts in midlife or later and shows no preference for women or for people with a family history of early-onset depression. Vascular depression causes more problems with memory and concentration, and it may respond less well to traditional antidepressant treatments.

Harry Finian's case, with his coronary disease triggering his first depressive episode at sixty, met this definition of vascular depression. At the time of Finian's first chest pains, the blood flow to his heart, and very likely to his brain, was reduced by his vascular disease. With surgery and medications the blood flow to both his heart and his brain presumably improved, and so did his depression. He never had a brain scan or a cerebral angiogram to assess the extent of cerebrovascular disease, but a couple of years ago he developed numbness in his left leg. His doctor told him he'd had a "mini-stroke" and started him on a blood thinner called Plavix, in addition to his daily aspirin. That helped, and the numbness went away. These facts about his illness only suggest the possibility of vascular depression. To establish this diagnosis would have required expensive brain-imaging techniques that were not available twelve years ago and even now are available only at a few research centers.

From Heart to Brain

Figure 8.1 shows the plausible pathways by which coronary disease leads to depression. Reading from lower right to upper left, this model assumes that atherosclerosis in the arteries of the heart may precede, coexist with, or follow the development of atherosclerosis in the arteries of the brain. Cardiovascular and cerebrovascular disease are the same weed in different patches of the garden. Sometimes heart disease provokes troubles in the brain, as when clots from the diseased heart vessels travel to the brain, causing strokes or mild transient ischemia or silent strokes. Heart attacks and arrhythmias and heart failure and chest pains and hypertension can also aggravate the effects of existing cerebrovascular disease by reducing the flow of blood to the brain. If your brain is already operating on marginal blood flow in some areas, one of these cardiac events could drop the level of blood flow to your limbic system even further. Surgical procedures like angioplasty and bypass surgery may also temporarily reduce cognitive functioning, possibly by disrupting blood flow to the brain.[3]

Sparked by heart attacks or severe chest pains or procedures to treat these problems, the sympathetic nervous system cranks out epinephrine and norepinephrine into a system that is already overstretched, making it work harder. Harry Finian's fear of death and his anxiety about facing pain and disability added to the demand on his cardiovascular system, most likely raising his blood pressure and heart rate, reducing blood flow further, exacerbating pain, and accelerating the whole process of atherosclerosis in his heart and his brain. For the first year after his angioplasty he couldn't think as fast on his feet, couldn't remember names as confidently as before, and at work couldn't concentrate on more than one task at a time. The common complaint of having trouble concentrating or remembering, when it persists beyond a few weeks, may reflect lower blood flow to any one of the many areas of the brain that serve short-term memory, such as the parietal cortex or the hippocampus.

If these problems are not quickly treated, the man or woman with the aching heart may in the weeks following a heart attack or severe chest pains be dominated by the casualties of caution: excessive avoidance of physical or sexual activity, repeated delays of returning to work, fear of overstimulation, cognitive slowing, and social withdrawal to dodge embarrassment. If recovery is not quick or assured, physical exhaustion and chronic stress then add to the burden of recovery. This combination of psychological, social, and physical burdens presents a formula for hopelessness, the kind that dragged Harry Finian into despair and kept him there for most of a year. Depression then becomes the psychological outcome of a series of events initiated by the emergence of heart disease onto a stage prepared for many years by the silent process of atherosclerosis in specific areas of the brain.

And the biology of this vascular depression is different from the biology of the depressed woman in her twenties whose brain arteries are as smooth as glass. The outward faces of the two depressions may look similar, but their biologies differ. We are beginning to see that vascular depression also calls for some innovative treatment approaches.

Clinical Tip 8.1: If you have heart disease, check on your brain.
Consider the possibility of vascular depression. If you're over fifty and develop depression after a heart attack or a heart procedure, even if you've had depression before, it may serve you well to get a thorough evaluation for vascular depression through your primary care physician. This may include an MRI scan of the brain, Doppler testing of the carotid arteries, or cognitive testing by a neuropsychologist, depending on your symptoms and your history. If your evaluation suggests the possibility of decreased blood flow in relevant parts of your brain, improvement of your depression may depend on regular exercise and improving your blood pressure, for example, in addition to an effective course of antidepressant medication or psychotherapy.

The vascular depression hypothesis, though the best biological explanation we have for depression following heart disease, is still, technically speaking, unproven. Conceivably, these patterns of scattered silent strokes

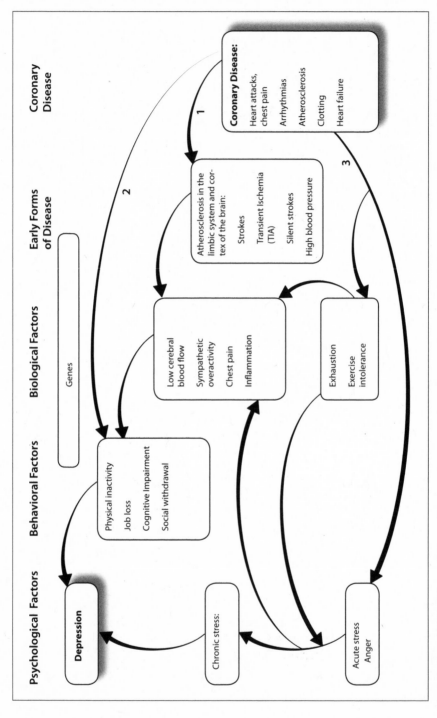

Figure 8.1. Plausible Pathways from Heart Disease to Depression

could result from some process other than decreased blood flow or atherosclerosis. Maybe these brain cells die as a part of the genetically programmed aging process, or fall victim to some toxic substance released by a still-undiscovered pathologic process. Though more common in people with late-onset depression, these silent ischemic lesions can be found on the brain images of a substantial number of elderly people who have no history of depression. Maybe the anatomic distributions of their lesions are different in important ways that have spared them from depression.

Closing the Loop

The other explanation for why people with no previous history of depression suddenly feel depressed after heart disease invokes a pathway from heart disease to behavior changes, pathway 2 in Figure 8.1. Heart disease pushes some people to change their approaches to daily life in ways that foster depression. They avoid doing anything strenuous, including activities that gave them pleasure. Burdensome medical bills may force cutbacks in hobbies. They may turn down invitations, put off trips, or postpone returning to work. These psychological shifts and behavior patterns designed to cope with heart disease exact a cost and may add up to a profound and persistent sense of loss, provoking clinical depression. A third alternative is that the heart disease poses such a threat over extended periods that anxiety and chronic stress wear down the central nervous system to the point of exhaustion and depression, pathway 3 in Figure 8.1. All three pathways may be at work at various times.

Because many factors contribute to the initiation of this cycle of stress, depression, and heart disease, it is often difficult to say where the cycle begins. The cycle suggested by Figures 7.4 and 8.1 operates through big loops and little loops. The biggest loop runs from depression to heart disease and back again, but that big loop may not establish itself until many years after the little loops have been hard at work. These little loops include such processes as depression fueling risky behaviors, which add to anxiety, which adds to depression. Or a genetically shy temperament may fuel sympathetic overdrive, which raises blood pressure, which reduces blood flow to the brain and raises anxiety, making the person withdraw more, which raises the risk for depression.[4]

We can enter any of these pathways at any point, and we can progress along these pathways in several directions simultaneously. That is, autonomic imbalance may raise my blood pressure at the same time that it makes me anxious and drives me to smoke more. Chest pain shuts down my willingness to push the lawn mower or do anything that would break a sweat, and my new status as resident couch potato in the long run makes my chest pain and heart disease worse. If I quit smoking the way my doctor and wife tell me to, how am I going to ease my nerves? Fudge ripple ice cream? That cools the burning in my chest, which is what I care about right now, more than the pounds it will put on my paunch. What can I do months later when my paunch hangs over my belt? I'm trapped and it's depressing as hell, which is bad for my autonomic nervous system, which is bad for my brain and bad for my heart. Round and round we go. There's gotta be more than one way out of here.

Defiant Hope

In 1932 when Norman Cousins was a ten-year-old schoolboy in New York City, his chronic cough led his doctor and his parents to send him away to a sanatorium in the Adirondack Mountains near Lake Saranac, New York. Sanitoriums at that time offered the best available treatment for tuberculosis but were places from which few children returned home. Norm immediately noticed that the ward culture in the children's TB unit divided into the kids who expected to survive and the kids who did not. The realists, the ones who did not expect to make it out, far outnumbered the optimists, but Norm gravitated immediately to the kids who defied the odds. "Nothing to me was more striking than the fact that far more optimists were able to conquer their illness than were the 'realists,'" he wrote many years later.[5] After a year far from home, struggling to defy the odds, Norman Cousins beat tuberculosis and went home with a lesson on the power of hope that he would soon forget in favor of more immediate boyish interests. But this lesson would serve him in at least two later struggles against life-threatening illness.

At fifty, Cousins, then editor of the weekly *Saturday Review* magazine and a father, husband, and avid tennis player in his spare time, began to feel persistent, severe back and joint pains. Nothing seemed to help, and after consulting multiple specialists, he finally learned that he had an unusual form of arthritis called ankylosing spondilitis. In 1964 there were no known cures for ankylosing spondilitis, and his doctors told him it would continue to worsen, tightening its stranglehold of inflammation and pain in a course of progressive debilitation. Ultimately he would die an early death from the immobility and pains imposed by the illness.

But, having wrestled with a gloomy prognosis early in life, and blessed with a defiant and hopeful temperament, Cousins put his journalistic skills to work and assigned members of his *Saturday Review* staff to help him find out more about this rare and terminal condition. He learned that his own immune system had turned against the cartilage in his joints, attacking the cartilage as though it were foreign tissue. The metaphorical importance of this fact impressed the editor in him, and he begun pursuing ways of closing the divide within his immune system. Instead of complying with the advice of doctors and nurses in the hospital, he took charge of many aspects of his care, such as when his blood was drawn, what he ate, and how many interruptions he had to put up with during the day and while asleep. He nearly got himself kicked out of the hospital, but his doctor sided with his unruly plans and paved the way for him to manage some aspects of his treatment. He took enormous doses of vitamin C by intravenous infusion and, believing that laughter is good medicine, he watched several hours daily of his favorite comedy movies. He found that "ten minutes of solid belly laughter would give me two hours of pain-free sleep. Since my illness ... [made] it painful even to turn over in bed, the practical value of laughter became a significant feature of treatment."[6]

Cousins's remarkable recovery from ankylosing spondilitis led him to write an article published in 1976 in the *New England Journal of Medicine*, an unusual achievement for a nonphysician. And in 1979 he published a book about his struggle, *Anatomy of an Illness*. The experience of recovering from this illness by taking charge of his own care so dominated his interests and passions from then on that within a few years Cousins abandoned his journalism career and his life in New York City to move with his wife to Los Angeles. In 1978 the college of medicine at UCLA offered him a professorship in the Department of Psychiatry and Behavioral Sciences. To take this position was a bold plunge for a sixty-three-year old journalist at the top of his profession, and he soon found that he had dived into foreign and not always friendly waters.

Outside of the enthusiasm of a select group within the UCLA Psychiatry Department, Cousins faced much skepticism among his new scientific colleagues at UCLA for his convictions about the power of the mind to overcome physical pathology, for his convictions that beliefs can shape biology. He found that compelling anecdotes such as his own don't count for much in a culture that reveres the double-blind, placebo-controlled clinical trial as the ultimate research test of a treatment's worth. Good stories would not persuade the skeptics. They wanted data.

In 1980, after just two years at UCLA and adhering to a particularly demanding travel schedule for speaking engagements, Cousins had a heart attack. Suddenly, instead of an esteemed public speaker in a suit, he was a very sick man in a gown alone in a coronary care unit. But drawing on his experiences and his own teachings about coping with illness, Cousins focused his efforts on warding off panic and helplessness. With the help of good care, several months of heart medications, and diligent participation in a cardiac rehabilitation program, by two months after the heart attack Cousins had recovered enough to walk four miles a day. He felt good, even though his cardiac assessment tests showed that his heart had only partly recovered, barely delivering enough oxygen to the mildly exercising heart. His cardiologist asked him how he "dealt with the depression that almost

---

Clinical Tip 8.2: If you develop heart disease, call on every resource that gives you hope and confidence. Of course this applies to coping with any serious illness, but because the biology of heart disease accelerates dramatically under the influence of depression and anxiety, it is especially helpful for people with heart disease to focus on cultivating hope and confidence during the first three to six months of recovery after a heart attack, bypass surgery, or an episode of severe chest pain. Friendship, prayer, exercise, good food, effective medication, useful information, psychotherapy, fun, cardiac rehabilitation, support groups, returning to work—whatever feeds your hope and confidence is good and essential treatment for heart disease, and good prevention for depression. It's hard to do too much of this kind of work.

---

universally affects people who have had heart attacks." Cousins told him that "the dominant emotion, not just at the time of the attack but during the critical period, was curiosity, a sense of challenge, and confidence.... I thought I had a great heart and that it was doing everything—and more— that anyone could ask of it."[7]

Cousins managed to avoid depression by arming himself with useful information about heart disease, by recruiting a team of doctors he trusted, and by leaning on his loving wife to help him with the complex recovery regimens of exercise, diet, and medications. Cousins was a born optimist who had successfully avoided clinical depression throughout a long and challenging life, but he had earned his confidence through hard-knocks experience in other arenas, and he put it to work fast when the heart attack hit. Once again he wrote about his troubles and triumphs. In 1983 he published an inspiring memoir of his experience recovering from his heart attack, *The Healing Heart: Antidotes to Panic and Helplessness*. He described in detail his negotiations with ambulance drivers, doctors, and family members about how to manage his care in ways that beat the threats of fear and depression.

This man's ability to overcome tuberculosis, severe arthritis, and severe heart disease, and then to write extensively about it, has made him an inspiring voice for patients and physicians. Norman Cousins' example for us is captured in the title of his final book, a memoir about his years at UCLA, *Head First: The Biology of Hope*, published in 1989, just a year before he finally died of heart disease at age seventy-five.

For those of us who do not have the temperament, experience, and brainpower of Norman Cousins, heart disease may bring with it a greater threat of depression. Now that we can understand the possible ways that this happens, we can develop effective treatment plans to reduce this threat.

CHAPTER 9

Tips for Better Care

The most powerful test of how well we understand an illness is how well we treat it. Sometimes, as in miracle cures and placebo responses, it's possible to treat an illness without understanding it. And all too often we understand an illness without being able to treat it effectively, as in many forms of cancer, AIDS in most of the world, and treatment-resistant tuberculosis. But, in general, throughout the history of modern medicine, the better we have understood complex illnesses, the more effective our treatments have become. And in the end, after the doctor's long-winded explanations of causes and effects, all the patient really cares about is how well the treatment works.

The good news for people with depression and heart disease is that for both illnesses, treatments work well. This chapter offers to these people, and to the clinicians who care for them, a guide to good treatment for depression and heart disease, beginning with how to lay the groundwork for treatment, and focusing then on common decisions patients with both conditions face.

As a reference point, the essentials of good treatment for depression by itself are available at several websites listed in Appendix G, "Resources for Treatment of Depression and Stress." And the essentials of good treatment for several forms of heart disease, apart from depression, are available at several websites listed in Appendix H, "Resources for Treatment of Heart Disease." This chapter focuses more narrowly on the treatment of the combination of these disorders.

Laying the Groundwork

Primary Care

Six of the Clinical Tips in the previous chapters relate to laying the groundwork for good treatment. A patient's ideal first step is to choose a good primary care doctor. More valuable to you than the cardiologist or the psychiatrist, the primary care doctor who sees you regularly over the years is the best person to help you spot risk factors early and to initiate treatments or preventive behavior changes long before you need to see a specialist. Your best hope for effective prevention lies in a sound relationship with your primary care doctor. And if you develop complicated depression or heart disease that requires a specialist, you'll need your primary care doctor to coordinate your care among several specialists over the years. So the first priority goes to the relationship with a primary care doctor.

Easy to say, and harder to do if you don't already work with a primary care doctor you like. But here are a few tips on how to find a primary care doctor who will manage both your depression and your heart disease. If any large primary care group practices are available to you, ask the practice manager or a nurse which doctors in the group particularly like treating depression and are good at it. Ask your friends and family in the area. Word of mouth is still our best initial way of finding good doctors. All primary care doctors treat heart disease at various levels of complexity, and most treat depression, at least initially. Ask for someone who will teach you about depression and heart disease, will prescribe antidepressant medications when you need them, and will refer you to good specialists if you need them. Visit several primary care doctors if necessary to find the doctor and the practice that suit your needs. Find out which psychiatrists and cardiologists your potential doctor usually refers to. Show your doctor what you've read. Find out what the staff can teach you about your depression and your heart disease. Talk to a nurse or an aid. In a fifteen-minute appointment you can often get the scoop and a feel for whether you could work with this doctor and this practice.

Though access to good primary care should be every individual's right, many of us lose our primary care doctors when our health-care plans restructure their benefits rules (sometimes an annual ritual), or when rising malpractice insurance rates cut our doctors out of business or raise them out of our financial reach. The whole U.S. health-care system needs radical surgery and resuscitation to preserve the role of the primary care clinician, but until it recovers, we will all have to scramble for the essential right to good primary care. If you can't find a primary care physician, but you have a relationship with a cardiologist or psychiatrist, make the best of your specialist to guide you in this process. For your purposes, a specialist or two is the next best thing to a good primary care physician.

Know Your Numbers

The second step toward better care is to learn your risks for depression and heart disease. This means gathering a few facts and a few numbers that describe your risks. This learning process, often thrust too late upon us by the surprise arrival in midlife of unwelcome symptoms, should begin early in adulthood, before habits and arteries have hardened. Until we learn what our risk factors are, we can't hope to manage our risks.

Begin with family history, as suggested in Clinical Tip 1.1. The exercise of drawing a family tree marked with the relevant illnesses often raises useful questions for prevention and treatment planning, pointing to patterns we miss in the more casual talk of family lore. Review the tree with your primary care doctor. Include conditions that are related to depression or heart disease, like alcoholism, anxiety, diabetes, high blood pressure, and obesity.

How old was Uncle Chester when he had that heart attack on the houseboat? If four men in my family had heart disease over the last three generations and three women had trouble with depression, then am I at risk for having both? After a careful review with your primary care doctor, you should come away with an impression of whether your family history contributes a low, medium, or high risk for depression, heart disease, or both. Gregory Hemingway's family tree in Chapter 4, Figure 4.1, shows that his family history contributed high risks for both conditions, pointing toward the need for aggressive prevention efforts and treatment by specialists when early conditions related to heart disease developed, such as high blood pressure.

Learning your risks for depression and heart disease, as suggested in Clinical Tips 3.2 and 3.4, means knowing your numbers. A few key numbers properly interpreted with the help of your physician provide a guide for how much preventive treatment you should consider before heart disease or depression develops. Men in their forties and women in their fifties should begin learning not only about their family histories but also about their cholesterol levels, blood pressure, body-mass index, glucose tolerance, physical activity patterns, number of episodes of major depression, and current severity of depressive symptoms.

You can use the flow diagram in Figure 7.4 to guide your discussion with your doctor about which risks apply to you and which numbers you need to know and follow. Knowing your numbers makes it harder to deny your risks. Most of us choose not to bother knowing these numbers until life forces them upon us. When I began working on this book in early 2002 at the age of fifty, I didn't need to know my numbers. I had no symptoms of either depression or heart disease, and I'd never had trouble with weight, smoking, or blood pressure. I figured I was clean. I vaguely remembered that once, six years earlier, my doctor had told me a random total cholesterol level had been high, over two hundred, but not high enough to require treatment. I felt fit, and my only addiction was to a good sweat at least twice a week playing soccer or tennis full tilt for an hour or two.

By the time I finished the first draft of Chapter 7 a year and a half later, well past my fifty-second birthday, I felt a rising uneasiness about my preaching in this book on the value of knowing your risks before symptoms strike. Stories about surprise heart attacks kept popping up on these pages. I started having more than a few conversations with myself about honesty, and finally I found my way to my family doctor for a check-up. Two days later he sent me my lab results sheet, with "start lipitor 10 mg/d" scrawled in the margin by the line that said "LDL cholesterol = 168." Yow! That number should be under 100. My total cholesterol was over 260 and should be under 200. Lipitor, or atorvastatin, is a common cholesterol-lowering drug. Me take medicine? But I play soccer and eat well. Yeah, man, cholesterol pills for you too. Join the heart-disease club.

My doctor also suggested I take advantage of a new commercial radiology organization in our area that was offering physicians free CT scans of the heart, a promotional deal to get us to recommend the $330 procedure to our patients. CT scans of the heart are still considered an elective prevention procedure and therefore are usually not covered by insurance. But I was eager to see this latest imaging machine, get something for nothing, and walk out with a clean bill on my heart. They shot the CT scan in a fifteen-minute appointment on my way to work one day, and two days later they called to tell me I have "calcium deposits in the left anterior descending artery" of my heart. I felt stunned. They gave me a score of 25, but the number I wanted was 0, which would mean I was "clean." The number 25 meant that I have mild to moderate calcification or plaque forming in that artery. A score over 100 means significant calcification, usually in several parts of several coronary arteries, and the radiologist reassured me he sees scores over 400 among the most advanced of his customers, so I was just getting started. He showed me my CT scan and pointed to a two-centimeter white streak, which he wryly called "the bone in your heart." It looked like a bone splinter, poised to stab. I will never think of my heart in the same way again.

A third number that popped up around this time was my C-reactive protein level (CRP), a measure of inflammation in the coronary arteries (briefly described in Chapter 6). My number, 1.01 mg/L, was above normal for men my age (<0.5 mg/L)—not severe, but high enough to jack my risk for heart disease up a notch. That is, if my elevated cholesterol by itself roughly doubles my risk for heart disease, adding the elevated CRP boosts my risk to roughly three times what it would have been if I had normal values for both numbers.[1] Thanks a lot. Now I know I have low-grade inflammation in my calcified left anterior descending coronary artery, bathed in plenty of LDL cholesterol. That's a bit of self-knowledge I could (and tried to) do without, but there it is now in plain numbers, and it's hard to deny.

The next stop on this self-exploration was an exercise treadmill test at the cardiologist's office. By now I was telling myself like a nervous coach that I would fly through this test, since it could hardly match the oxygen demands of an hour and a half of hard soccer or tennis. But no, this test came back with a reading of "possibly abnormal" due to the suggestion of some strain, "ST depressions" on my electrocardiogram during the highest level of exercise. That couldn't be, I thought. I'd felt nothing but strong during the treadmill test. My heart works fine under greater demands than this little treadmill. Was this just a laboratory goose chase? They told me to come back for another round. To my relief, the next level of testing, a stress echocardiogram, done two days after my mother died of a stroke at eighty-two, turned out to be normal, and that ended the evaluation process.

But not before the cardiologist showed me what he likes about the way the walls of my heart flap in toward each other with each pump, and he said the "possibly abnormal" readings on the earlier test didn't mean anything. But, he said, even though my heart functions well, I do have the early signs of coronary disease and I should take a cholesterol-lowering drug and aspirin every day for the rest of my life. These numbers and the heart scan were no false alarms from the laboratory. They certified me as a true heart-disease patient.

Two years ago I had no intention of serving so soon as an example in my own book, but now these numbers and that "bone" in my heart have changed the way I look, inwardly at least. They've added taking pills (atorvastatin and aspirin) to my morning shaving ritual. They may also have added length to my life. We'll see.

Pick Your Targets

Once you've established a relationship with a primary care doctor and identified your risk factors for depression and heart disease, the next step is to pick your targets for prevention and treatment. Picking your targets or setting priorities for treatment is often guided by your access to treatment resources. Does your insurance cover cardiac rehabilitation or psychotherapy? Will your doctor or nurse share information about treatments? What specialists can you see?

Pain or fear often lends urgency to one factor over another. People in distress may underestimate their resources and feel unnecessarily helpless when resources may be around the corner. It helps to talk with health professionals and other patients with similar problems to find out what's available to you. On the other hand, if you live in a rural area, you may not have easy access to mental health specialists or cardiologists, so target problems that you can treat with what resources you have.

If you have multiple risk factors, start by picking the one or two targets that you can most easily improve. For example, if you're lucky enough to be good at losing weight, focus all your efforts on achieving a target of moderate weight loss. That may eliminate your need for blood pressure medication or diabetes medication, and that weight loss will make it easier to increase your physical activity level. Or, it may be easier and quicker for you to lower your blood pressure with a medication than to lose weight. If that's true, lower your blood pressure first. I chose to start lowering my cholesterol with a daily medication because the medication is easier than a diet, I'm more reliable about pills than about food, and my insurance pays for the medication. If it's easy, start there. Once you improve in one area, it becomes easier to reduce the other risk factors.

Pick your targets and be patient. It took decades to build these processes that contribute to depression and heart disease, and it usually takes several years—not days or weeks—to reverse them. Give yourself several years of concentrated effort to lower your risks.

Special Treatment Decisions

Though most of the treatment decisions faced by doctors and their patients with depression and heart disease follow in a straightforward way from the guidelines for treating either disorder alone, a few decisions can be tricky and deserve special attention. The following recommendations rest on the best published clinical experience, expert opinions, and clinical research, but relatively few rigorously designed studies have looked at the effectiveness of treatments in people with both depression and heart disease.

The options for treatment of coronary heart disease boil down to three types of approaches: bypass surgery, including angioplasty and stents; change of risk-related behaviors; and medications. If you have a history of depression or develop depression during these cardiac treatments, you face some additional treatment decisions that could improve your chances of doing well.

Bypass Surgery, Angioplasty, and Stents

One in five people develop major depression within weeks after the surgical correction of narrowed coronary arteries. And depression increases the risk for needing a second corrective procedure within five years. That is, the same or a new narrowing of the coronary artery is more likely to happen in depressed people than in those who are not depressed. And for many people depression soon after a heart attack or unstable angina doubles or triples the risk for dying from coronary disease.[2] For these three reasons (if dodging the misery of depression is not compelling enough by itself), it's a good idea to do what you can to avoid depressions after cardiac procedures. I recommend to people who have a history of depression that they consider taking an antidepressant medication, or psychotherapy for depression, in a preventive manner for at least the first six months after the cardiac procedure to protect against a recurrence of depression. Until careful studies examine the effectiveness of taking preventive antidepressants to improve cardiac outcomes, the justification for this approach will rest on clinical judgment about the benefits of potentially preventing an episode of depression during this period of increased cardiac vulnerability. For people who can't take or choose not to take antidepressant medication, other options for preventing depression may be equally effective, such as psychotherapy, exercise, and light therapy.[3]

Behavior Change

One of the most important riddles modern medicine has yet to crack for the benefit of heart disease and many other chronic illnesses is how to change high-risk health behaviors for large numbers of people. Sustained behavior change is tough for most of us, and, in general, doctors in the United States report low success rates in helping their patients quit smoking, lose weight, or exercise regularly.

However, a group of researchers has shown that the principles of one of the most effective smoking-cessation methods also apply with promising success rates to changing other health-related behaviors, such as physical inactivity, unsafe sex, overeating, and even cocaine abuse. This "stages of change" method, originally developed by James Prochaska and his colleagues and described in their inspiring self-help book *Changing for Good*, has been adopted by the Centers for Disease Control and Prevention, the National Cancer Institute, and the National Health Service of Great Britain in a wide range of programs for reducing risky behaviors. These researchers have shown that patients, on their own and with the help of clinicians, can make sustained behavior changes that improve their health outcomes. Doctors, along with their patients with depression and heart disease, will find their efforts at changing high-risk behaviors more rewarding if they follow the guidelines spelled out in *Changing for Good*.

Briefly, the process works like this. Begin by establishing your stage of readiness for change. Ask yourself if you are (a) denying the problem exists (precontemplation), (b) thinking about changing but not in the next six months (contemplation), (c) planning on changing within the next six months (planning), (d) taking action toward changing a behavior (action), or (e) maintaining the changed behavior (maintenance). Then the task is to figure out how to move to the next stage of readiness for change, rather than jump ahead to quitting the behavior. For each transition to the next stage the effective techniques vary. Startling an alcoholic into contemplating sobriety requires a different set of techniques than does helping him bypass the liquor store. Persuading a healthy fifty-two-year-old to go get his cholesterol checked requires a different strategy than getting him to stop eating pork chops and chitlins.

Once you choose the behavior you want to change, look at the pros and cons of changing to the new behavior (which might be, for example, smoking only half a pack a day or doing Jane Fonda video workouts twice a week for half an hour) using a measure called the decision balance. Success at behavior change is usually tied to the length of the list of pros for the new behavior on the decision-balance measure. The more arguments you can mount for the new behavior, the more likely you are to achieve the change and maintain it. Finally, motivational interviewing is the counseling approach for helping people translate their particular set of arguments for and against a behavior change into a treatment plan that works. Though some steps can be accomplished on your own, most people find that it's most efficient and least frustrating to work with a counselor who is familiar with this approach to changing health-related behaviors.

Cardiac Rehabilitation

If you've had a heart attack or unstable angina, somebody has probably talked to you about cardiac rehabilitation, the most commonly prescribed approach to rapid change of cardiac risk behaviors. These rehabilitation programs combine exercise regimens, diet changes, medication adjustments, cardiovascular monitoring, and education about heart disease for two to four months at varying levels of intensity. In spite of many studies showing that an organized program of daily outpatient cardiac rehabilitation treatment improves the recovery from heart attacks and unstable angina, fewer than half of all people for whom it is recommended take advantage of cardiac rehabilitation.[4] For some people, rehabilitation is not covered by insurance; for others, the program takes too much effort or time, or it's too far away.

For those who also suffer from depression, cardiac rehabilitation serves as good therapy, both physically and emotionally. Rehabilitation programs reduce fears about heart disease, provide group support, and reduce distress through graded levels of exercise training in safe conditions. Some provide relaxation training and stress-management classes.

But cardiac rehabilitation should not be considered a substitute treatment for major depression. Most rehab programs do not assess depression symptoms or diagnose mental disorders, and they do not provide medications specifically for depression. Most people with major depression that persists for several weeks after a cardiac event need treatment for the depression by their primary care doctor, a mental health specialist, or a cardiologist, in addition to whatever benefits they reap from cardiac rehab. On the other hand, depressed people with heart disease need rehabilitation programs perhaps more than anyone. They may resist attending rehab more stubbornly than others do, but, once engaged, depressed people are likely to reap dual benefits from cardiac rehab for both depression and heart disease. The package of frequent supportive social contact, regular exercise, reduced pain, and stress-management training proves a good combination for recovering from depression, as well as from a heart attack.

Diet

If you have depression and heart disease, the best thing you can do for your diet is eat plenty of fish or take omega-3 fatty acid supplements. Fish oil, which is so rich in omega-3 fatty acids, is good for the heart and good for the brain. The American Heart Association now includes details on fish and omega-3 in its dietary recommendations for heart disease (*www. americanheart.org*; search Omega-3). And for those with a talent for dietary discipline, the Cretan Mediterranean diet, which is high in olive oil, whole grains, vegetables, beans, and nuts, has proven to reduce heart attacks and strokes within four years.[5]

Though we have known for thirty years about lower rates of heart disease in countries whose populations eat a lot of fish, such as Japan, Iceland, Korea, and Mediterranean Europe, only in the late 1990s did we learn about a similar association between depression and fish intake around the world. Countries where people consume large amounts of fish generally report lower rates of depression than countries where people consume little fish, such as Germany, Hungary, and New Zealand. A few studies have shown that within a population, those with lower levels of omega-3 fatty acids have higher scores for depressive symptoms.[6]

The key ingredient in fish oil for both depression and heart disease is a group of fatty acids called omega-3 fatty acids, consisting primarily of eicosapentaenoic acid (EPA) and docosahexaenoic acid (DHA). Because we can neither pronounce nor synthesize these molecules, we must abbreviate and eat them. In that sense they are like vitamins.

We need EPA and DHA to make the membranes of most cells, particularly nerve and muscle cells in the brain and heart. When we take in too little of these omega-3 fatty acids over long stretches of time, the membranes of these cells function less well and the cells survive less long. The central nervous system and the cardiovascular system wear down faster and illnesses develop sooner.

Careful studies of omega-3 fatty acids as treatments for heart disease have shown benefits by reducing arrhythmias and sudden death, reducing triglyceride levels, and reducing the rate of atherosclerotic plaque growth. Studies of omega-3 fatty acids as treatments for depression are in their infancy, but a handful of small trials have shown promising effects of omega-3 treatments on depressive symptoms and relapse rates in depression and bipolar disorder. Still, we don't yet know the answers to some critical questions about the use of omega-3 for depression, such as what the necessary doses and durations are, whether omega-3 works best as a supplement or as the primary treatment, and whether it works in severe depressions, as well as in mild ones. Most studies have examined the effectiveness of 600–1000 mg of omega-3 fatty acids (EPA and DHA) per day, the equivalent of one supplement capsule a day.[7]

How much fish or omega-3 supplement should you eat? The American Heart Association recommends three dosing levels, depending on the goal: (a) to reduce the chance of developing coronary disease in those who don't have it, eat fish twice a week; (b) for those who have coronary disease, eat fish every day or take one omega-3 supplement prescribed by your physician; and (c) to lower triglycerides, take two to four grams of omega-3 fatty acids a day by supplements. Most supplements contain about one gram of omega-3 fatty acids. A one-month supply costs from twelve to twenty-five dollars, depending on dose and brand. For most people, taking one capsule of omega-3 supplement a day will benefit both the depression and the heart disease. Though you don't need a prescription for omega-3 supplements, talk with your physician about dose and brand, because too much omega-3 can cause belching or, occasionally, bleeding.

If tuna and salmon don't grab your fancy, try herring, sardines, blue-fish, or mackerel. If you can't stomach fish at all, you can get your omega-3 in venison or buffalo steaks. Vegans can rely on canola oil, olive oil, walnuts, and purslane. A quarter of a cup of walnuts (one ounce) gives you as much omega-3 as three ounces of salmon. If you like walnuts on your salmon, you might double the benefit.

One final point about diet for people with depression and heart disease. Losing weight ranks among the toughest behavior changes. For most of us losing weight is long, slow, frustrating work. Since there's no quick fix for obesity (even weight loss with the help of bariatric or gastric bypass surgery takes about a year from start to a stable lower weight), we rely on discipline, tenacity, and patience as much as on any formal program or diet to achieve a stable lower weight. Losing weight is hard enough to do when we have all our wits about us, and it's no job for the depressed mind. Depression can sabotage the best-laid plans for weight loss, particularly if you tend to eat or drink more when depressed. The depressed mind is famous for shifting moods and behaviors, giving up easily, running out of patience in the face of frustration, seeing oneself as ugly, and predicting failure. If any of those mind tricks sound familiar, before you launch into an ambitious diet or weight-loss program, make sure you've treated your depression as fully as possible and stay on whatever antidepressant treatment works for you while you're losing weight.

For most people SSRI antidepressants do not cause weight gain or interfere with weight loss. Bupropion is also a good antidepressant for people who want to lose weight. Topiramate, an anticonvulsant and mild mood stabilizer, actually promotes weight loss and may help keep your moods stable while you're dieting. On the other hand, mirtazapine and some tricyclic antidepressants (amitryptiline, imipramine) promote weight gain and should be avoided while you're dieting to lose weight.

Vitamins

There is some evidence that a combination of vitamins B_6, B_{12}, and folate lowers homocysteine, which reduces risk for vascular disease in general.[8]

Exercise

Next to losing weight, increasing physical activity may be the hardest health behavior to sustain. But for people with depression and heart disease, exercise is like omega-3: You can hit two targets with one bullet, treat two ailments with one medicine. What's good for your heart is good for your brain.

And we're not talking about marathons or muscle-beach contests. We're talking about the equivalent of three half hours of brisk walking each week to get started. You don't even have to change your clothes or break a sweat. If you're not doing that much exercise, you're cheating your heart and your brain. More may be better, but only up to a point. And it's never too late. No matter how long you have dodged exercise or how old you are, exercise can reduce your risk for heart disease.

For your heart, exercise sets the range of vascular tone throughout the system, from the largest (your heart) to the smallest vessels (the tiny arterioles where the oxygen diffuses across arteriole walls and into the tissues). Think of exercise as a tune-up for various levels of demand on your cardiovascular system, a drill that calls into action the coordination of hormones, nerves, and the muscles in the vessel walls. The drill also tunes up the immune system and the limbic system. Once finely tuned, the rises in adrenalin, cortisol, and endorphins account for the transient good feeling, the runner's high, that comes with exercise, often overriding the aches and the fatigue.

For your brain, in addition to that transient good feeling, exercise promotes neurogenesis, or nerve-cell regeneration, in the hippocampus of the limbic system, the part of the brain that shrinks under prolonged stress or depression. Exercise restructures this part of the limbic system in a way that improves the functioning of the whole system. When you walk or jog or swim, you may be building brain "muscle" as well as body muscle, particularly if you've had major depression. In this sense, for many people regular exercise works as an antidepressant both immediately (within minutes and lasting hours) and over the long run (lasting weeks to months).

Studies of exercise as a treatment for heart disease show a beneficial effect both for the prevention of coronary disease and for the improvement of existing coronary disease. Studies of exercise as a treatment for depression have focused mostly on mild to moderate depression and suggest that sustained regular exercise reduces depressive symptoms as much as psycho-therapy or antidepressant medication does, and that exercise reduces the risk of relapse.[9]

The level of exercise required to reduce risk for heart disease is about the same as the level required to reduce symptoms of depression. Thirty minutes of vigorous walking three times a week is a good goal to start with for people who usually do nothing that would pass for exercise (about half the U.S. population). Beyond that level the benefits increase with increasing duration and frequency, up to a point. Most of the benefits can be achieved by thirty to sixty minutes of daily vigorous walking or light jogging. Any combination of exercise types and durations will do, such as several fifteen-minute walks, so do whatever is most convenient. Marathon runners or walkers don't do any better than 5K runners or walkers in the race against heart disease or depression, so you can thumb your nose at them.[10]

Medications

The first important point about medications is that no common cardiac medication causes depression, and in general, people with depression and heart disease do not have to avoid any specific cardiac medications. The long-held misconception among many doctors that beta-blockers like propranolol or atenolol cause depression was based on sloppy science and has been refuted a number of times over the last few years.[11] But prescribing habits, even sloppy ones, die hard, so it will take some effort to correct this habit of avoiding beta-blockers in depressed patients with heart disease. On the contrary, beta-blockers are good for the depressed patient with heart disease. Beta-blockers prevent the autonomic instability, the excessive adrenalin surges (overreactions in our sympathetic nervous systems), and the loss of fine regulation of blood pressure, heart rate, and heart-rate variability that often follow heart attacks, and that are also features of the autonomic dysregulation noted in severe depressive episodes.

The second important point about medications is that no antidepressant medications cause heart disease. However, because of side effects, some antidepressant medications are better than others for heart disease. For example, the selective serotonin reuptake inhibitors (SSRIs) are safe and effective for the treatment of major depression in people with coronary disease. In fact, a few studies suggest that SSRIs may protect against heart disease, but more research will be needed to establish the validity of that protective effect.[12]

In contrast, another group of antidepressants, the tricyclic antidepressants, though they do not cause heart disease, may make existing heart disease worse. If you have heart disease, and particularly if you've had a heart attack in the past year, you should avoid the tricyclic antidepressants, such as amitryptiline, nortryptiline, imipramine, or desipramine. Tricyclic antidepressants may make the heart slip into arrhythmias (irregular heart rhythms) during the period of months when the heart muscle is irritable as it recovers from the recent injury of the heart attack. This effect of antidepressants on arrhythmias was discovered in the 1980s when a large treatment trial of drugs designed specifically to reduce arrhythmias found that instead they increased the risk of dying of sudden death when taken in the months after a heart attack. Tricyclic antidepressants, which are chemically related to these anti-arrhythmic drugs, have this same paradoxical arrhythmic effect during this period of heart-muscle irritability. So, in general, avoid tricyclic antidepressants if you have coronary disease or cardiac arrhythmias.[13]

Which antidepressants are best for the treatment of depression in heart disease? As Table 9.1 shows, any of the SSRIs (sertraline, citalopram, escitalopram, paroxetine, and fluoxetine) are safe and effective, based on more than ten years of clinical experience, FDA monitoring, and a few studies. However, one SSRI, sertraline, has been studied in a large and scientifically rigorous manner for its safety and efficacy in patients with recent heart attacks or unstable angina. And this medication has also proven safe and effective for treating or preventing depression in a few other studies of patients with heart disease or stroke. Because we know more about sertraline in heart disease than about the other SSRIs, and because it's among the cheapest of these expensive drugs, I often recommend sertraline as a good medication to begin with for treating depression in a person with heart disease.

One cautionary note may provide guidance in the search for an effective antidepressant in people who have "vascular depression," as described in Chapter 8. The likelihood of responding to an antidepressant diminishes with increasing numbers of cardiac risk factors, so treatment response may

Table 9.1. Effects of Specific Antidepressants on Heart Disease

Class	Cardiac Effects	Treatment Considerations
Serotonin Reuptake Inhibitors		
Citalopram (Celexa)	May reduce clotting	May need to reduce doses of other blood thinners
Escitalopram (Lexapro)		
Sertraline (Zoloft)		
Paroxetine (Paxil)		
Fluoxetine (Prozac)		
Miscellaneous		
Venlafaxine (Effexor)	At doses >300 mg/d, may raise blood pressure	Avoid high doses or monitor blood pressure in patients with high blood pressure
Mirtazepine (Remeron)	Weight gain	Avoid in patients with diabetes or obesity
Duloxetine (Cymbalta)		Possibly more effective than others against physical pain
Bupropion (Wellbutrin)		
Tricyclics		
Amitryptiline (Elavil)	Arrhythmias after heart attacks	Avoid in all patients with coronary disease or at risk for developing coronary disease
Nortryptiline (Pamelor)		
Imipramine (Tofranil)		
Desipramine (Norpramin)		

require reducing some of those risk factors as well as unusual persistence to find the right combination of treatments.[14]

Several antidepressants cause side effects that should be avoided in people with heart disease. Venlafaxine, when taken at high doses (above 300 mg/d), may raise blood pressure, exacerbating heart disease or making the management of high blood pressure more difficult. Mirtazapine makes some people gain weight, so don't bother with this medication if you're trying to lose weight. On the other hand, if depression has robbed you of your appetite and made you lose too much weight, mirtazapine can help both your depression and your weight loss.

And finally, if anxiety bothers you while you're depressed, bupropion may make your anxiety initially worse. It's a stimulating antidepressant for many people, and it sometimes makes people more anxious during the first few weeks they take it. On the other hand, if your depression saps your energy and drags you down, bupropion may be an activating medication for you and good for your heart disease. It carries the double benefit of being effective for both depression and smoking cessation, so I often prescribe it for smokers with depression and heart disease. It is also the antidepressant least likely to cause sexual dysfunction, so it's a good choice for people who have had sexual side effects from other antidepressants or for people whose heart disease interferes with sexual functioning.

Drug Interactions

With a few exceptions, the medications that are commonly used for heart disease can be taken with the medications that are commonly used for depression. People with coronary disease often take blood thinners that reduce the tendency to form clots, medications like aspirin, warfarin (Coumadin), or clopidogrel (Plavix). Since SSRI antidepressants may also, to a mild degree, reduce the tendency to form clots, it's possible that SSRIs may add to the blood-thinning or anti-clotting effect of these medications. Though not a common problem, this interaction is worth knowing about. It does not usually mean that these medications cannot be taken together at all, but doses may need to be adjusted. If easy bruising or bleeding becomes a problem while on this combination of medications, blood tests of the clotting process can measure the severity of the problem, and dose adjustments can fix it.

Drug Side Effects

Antidepressants, particularly SSRIs, may cause a loss of interest in sex or interfere with sexual functioning. The severity of this side effect varies widely from person to person and may occur with one SSRI but not another. Because both depression and heart disease may also interfere with sexual function, it can be tricky to figure out whether the medication or the underlying illness is causing the problem. The answer usually comes with the details of the timing of the sexual dysfunction or by temporarily stopping the antidepressant medication for a few days and then restarting it. If it's a side effect of the drug, the sexual dysfunction disappears within days of stopping it and it returns when you resume the medication.

Consider the middle-aged man whose depression turns sex from a pleasure to a chore. He takes an SSRI for the depression and promptly loses his ability to have sex at all. This man, if he's the common American man or Bob Dole, is likely to ask his doctor for sildanefil, or Viagra, and expect to get it. But erectile dysfunction, or difficulty maintaining an erection, may be a side effect of the SSRI or an effect of depression or a sign of poor blood flow to the penis because of peripheral vascular disease. The good doctor will evaluate this man's risk for heart disease before writing the sildanefil prescription, since sildanefil can make heart disease worse and should not be taken by people with active coronary disease.[15]

Statin drugs, such as simvastatin and atorvastatin, can cause aches and pains in muscles and joints. Depression is also famous for causing aches and pains, so when you're trying to ease these aches, consider both depression and statins as possible contributing factors. With adequate physician monitoring, stopping the statin drug or lowering the dose for several weeks may clarify whether the aches are a side effect of the drug or a feature of the depression. Contrary to the occasional rumor, cholesterol-lowering drugs do not raise the risk for depression or suicide.

Alternatives to Medications

For people who can't tolerate, don't like, or don't respond to drugs, there are a number of effective alternatives for treating both depression and heart disease. For depression, the alternatives for which we have evidence of effectiveness include cognitive therapy, interpersonal therapy, exercise, light therapy, omega-3 fatty acid or fish-oil diet, and electroconvulsive therapy, or ECT. For heart disease, the alternatives to medications are surgery (including angioplasty), exercise, and diet.[16]

Dean Ornish

Dean Ornish's "Program for Reversing Heart Disease" consists of intensive training in diet, stress reduction, and exercise. Several studies have shown the Ornish program can reverse the progression of coronary atherosclerosis, but so far only a select group of people have been willing to commit themselves to such a "boot-camp experience" to change the way they live.[17] Most people find that they need to use more than one approach over several years to establish control over either depression or heart disease.

Psychotherapy

In the supermarket of psychotherapies available to many Americans, it's harder to find the right brand of psychotherapy than it is to find the right brand of rye bread in the grocery store. But if you know what you're looking for, the search narrows to a manageable number of options. Use your primary care physician as your shopping guide in your local area. Word of mouth is still the surest way to find the best psychotherapists in your area, and you may have to try several to find a good fit. Because of their medical orientation, psychiatrists who do psychotherapy or psychologists who practice in medical settings (clinics or hospitals) are best suited to provide psychotherapy for depression in the context of heart disease.

Two forms of psychotherapy, cognitive therapy for depression and interpersonal therapy for depression, have proven in rigorous scientific studies over the past twenty years to be as effective as antidepressant medications for the relief of depressive symptoms and for recovery from a major depressive episode. Try to find a mental health specialist who can provide either of these forms of psychotherapy. They both require eight to sixteen sessions for most cases, which translates into an hour once a week for two to four months. Psychotherapy teaches you skills for managing your depression that reduce the risk for relapse well after you stop attending sessions. Many experts feel that the best treatment for major depression is the combination of antidepressant medication and psychotherapy for depression. .

Psychotherapy is also a powerful tool for managing the behavioral aspects of heart disease. Use psychotherapy, including group therapy, to improve your adherence to complex medication regimens, to lower your blood pressure through stress-reduction techniques, to lower your weight, and to reduce your need for medications for chest pain.[18] To illustrate this process, Appendix I, "Summary of a Course of Cognitive Therapy in a Fifty-One-Year-Old Man with Depression and Coronary Disease," summarizes the treatment of a man with major depression and coronary disease using a combination of cognitive therapy, antidepressant medications, and standard cardiac treatments.

Light Therapy

Like exercise and omega-3 supplements, bright light therapy is an underused alternative for the treatment of major depression. It requires buying a lamp for about two hundred dollars and sitting close to it for half an hour each morning. If two hundred dollars seems like a stiff price for a bright lamp, think of it as the price of one or two months of name-brand antidepressant medication. Studies suggest that light therapy can effectively treat moderate major depression either as a substitute for antidepressant medications or as an adjunct for people who only get partly well with medications.[19]

ECT

Electroconvulsive therapy is the most rapid and effective treatment for severe major depression. People whose depression has made them bedridden, unable to care for themselves, or acutely suicidal usually begin to function within a week or ten days of starting ECT. And ECT is safe for people with heart disease, so it is particularly important to consider ECT for people whose severe depression interferes with the acute care of their heart disease.[20]

Pets

Though the number of studies is small, there is plenty of folk wisdom and some evidence that owning a pet, particularly a dog, is good for your heart. And pets may buffer the effects of chronic illnesses, reducing the likelihood of depression.[21]

Herbs

Over the past generation, Western medicine has begun to learn from Chinese medicine new ways of understanding and treating illness. Diagnoses and treatments in Chinese medicine are less constrained by anatomic distinctions than in Western medicine, so a single herb may treat both the heart and distress. For example, Section 2 in Chapter 14 of the Materia Medica in *Chinese Herbal Medicine* is called "Formulas That Nourish the Heart and Calm the Spirit." These formulas include sour jujube seed, iron filings, arborvitae seed, and mimosa tree bark. The enduring power of these remedies suggests that, as has occurred with acupuncture, Western scientific investigations will soon make scientific sense of their curative properties.[22]

In the past twenty years the number of treatment options for depression and heart disease, as well as their safety, their affordability, and their efficacy, have multiplied. And compared to twenty years ago, many more people make use of these new treatments. That's the good news.

The bad news is that, even in the United States and Europe, where access to health care is the best in the world, fewer than half the people who need it get adequate treatment for either heart disease or depression.[23] And for people who have both heart disease and depression, the chance of receiving good treatment for either illness is even lower than if they had one or the other illness alone. On a large public health scale we have not yet figured out practical ways to get good treatment to the majority of people with both heart disease and depression.

This is just one reason why the health-care system in the United States sorely needs fixing.[24] But while we wait for the health-policy wonks in Washington to invent a better system, how can we find good treatment? In many respects the obstacles we face as individual patients trying to achieve good results through treatments for depression and heart disease parallel the obstacles faced by public health approaches to any common disabling chronic illness. We have to find out as early as possible if we are at risk, change our high-risk behaviors sufficiently and for long enough to prevent the development or progression of each illness, and find effective treatments and continue them long enough to reduce the risks for progression of each illness. This approach to chronic conditions requires a different set of attitudes, skills, and resources than does the usual approach to acute illnesses, such as pneumonia or a broken bone. Unfortunately, during the twentieth century we built our health-care system—hospitals, clinics, health insurance, training programs—to concentrate first and best on managing acute illnesses. It takes extra effort and savvy by both the doctor and the patient to make this system serve the care of conditions like depression and heart disease, which demand that we try to prevent life-threatening acute events, as well as manage underlying chronic conditions.

For incurable conditions like coronary disease and the more severe forms of depression, the best treatment is prevention. But worldwide the number of people and the proportion of the population developing these two illnesses continues to grow each decade, suggesting that globally we have made no overall progress in the prevention of either depression or heart disease. In spite of unprecedented public health campaigns for heart-disease prevention in the United States, the gains we've made by cutting smoking rates and cholesterol levels during the last forty years of the twentieth century have been outweighed by the obesity and diabetes epidemics of the 1980s and 1990s. The number of people developing coronary disease in the United States continues to rise. Depression rates in the United States have risen steadily since 1936. The lucky minority of people with heart disease who get good treatment now live longer, and those who get treatment for depression function better, but the result is that more people live longer with these two disorders now than ever before.[25]

I want you to leave this chapter with a brighter view of the possibilities for survival, a better command of the options for thriving in spite of two tough health conditions. Of course, to thrive requires teamwork and knowledge and persistence and a willingness to try new combinations of treatments. The benefits come gradually. A bit of luck helps. Treating depression and heart disease can be hard work, especially in the beginning, but the alternatives—suffering, disability, or early death—make the work of treatment, in the balance, the better way to go.

CHAPTER 10

A Call for Change

The stories in this book of Tom Geraci, Paula Volk, Ted O'Reilly, Gregory Hemingway, Gloria Wachuka, and others dramatize their individual struggles against the insidious and sometimes vicious cycle of stress, depression, and heart disease. These stories remind us that, one by one, we too can find ways to break the cycle and make treatments work for us. We can do a lot individually to improve the way we take care of our minds and our bodies, but the combination of depression and heart disease is a problem not just for a few unlucky people. Depression and heart disease are problems for our society—common, costly, and treatable problems. They emerged in the twentieth-century United States as "social diseases" that have flourished in response to environmental shifts in diet, diminishing physical activity, social fragmentation, substance abuse, and the stresses of urban living. The social dimensions of depression and heart disease cry out for broad-reaching remedies in the way our society delivers health care. The stories in this book testify about struggles within a health-care system that fails us in costly, often crucial, ways. These failures demand systemwide change before too many of them break the bank.

But what can be done and who will do the changing? In the last chapter we talked about what patients and their doctors can do. So much for the little guys. What can the big guys do, the ones with the clout—the organizational heads, the policy makers, the legislators? One of the strongest voices calling for high-impact remedies in our health-care system is the Institute of Medicine. In its visionary 2001 report, *Crossing the Quality Chasm: A New Health System for the 21st Century*, the IOM identified the major flaws in the current structure of the cost-crazy U.S. health-care delivery system and concluded that we need more than a tune-up. We need an overhaul, and the institute's report designs the overhaul.[1]

To better care for the chronically ill and to prevent the growing burden of chronic illnesses, this report argues that we have to reinvent our system of care using new technologies that allow us to manage large databases on large groups of patients with a given problem or illness, monitoring the effectiveness of our care and systematically improving our deficiencies. We need changes at almost every level of the system: patients, doctors, clinics, managed-care organizations, insurance-reimbursement policies, advocacy groups like the American Heart Association and the American Psychiatric Association, priorities for federal research, and national standards for medical training.

In a 2003 report, *Priority Areas for National Action: Transforming Health Care Quality*, the IOM ranked improving care for major depression and ischemic heart disease among the top twenty priorities for action in the transformation of health care.[2] This call for changes in how we as a society care for large numbers of people with chronic illnesses in the United States suggests to me that improving the care of people with depression and heart disease, in particular, depends on local and national health-policy leaders implementing at least six major changes in our current system of care. Imagine how a new health system in this twenty-first century might take care of those of us with depression and heart disease. Without these changes, our future care will look too much like the inadequate care of the past.

1. Integrate Mental Health Services into Primary Care Practices

In our current system, the treatment of your mental disorder usually takes place apart from the treatment of your physical disorder. Your depression usually requires you to go to a different clinic or office from your primary care doctor and see a different clinician on a different day, often paying through a different insurance plan than the one that pays for your heart disease. No wonder only one in three referrals to mental health specialists actually result in a completed visit! And when you do follow up, records of the treatment of your mind rarely find their way to the records of the treatment of your body. These obstacles not only waste your time and money, but also make it so inconvenient for you and your doctor to pursue mental health treatment that both of you avoid the effort for as long as you can. If your primary care doctor does treat your depression, she or he will often bill your insurance company for "fatigue" or "insomnia," instead of "depression" in order to get paid, because many managed-care companies won't pay primary care physicians for treating mental illnesses. That financial disincentive amounts to a not-so-subtle directive to the primary care doctor to refer away all mental disorders, to misdiagnose them for billing purposes, or to ignore them.

What's the solution? When primary care group practices integrate mental health specialists into their teams, they go a long way toward closing the gap for the patient and the physician. A few integrated practices exist, but it's a marvel of tradition and inertia that more HMOs, managed-care plans, and large group practices have not adopted this integrated model. When you see your primary care doctor and a mental health specialist in the same office or organization, it's easy and it makes sense, like having a heart and a brain in the same body. One site, one group, one chart, one billing system, and a team whose members talk to each other about your treatment plan. Integrating mental health care into primary care is essential to improving our dismal rates of effective treatment for depression in patients with heart disease. If you have depression and heart disease and can choose where you go, shop for a practice that integrates mental health care into primary care. If you run a primary care practice, hire a mental health specialist or two. It's good for your patients, good for society, and good for your business.[3]

2. Establish Guidelines for Screening for Depression in Patients at Risk for Coronary Disease

If you have heart disease, do you expect your doctor to check for depression symptoms as part of the routine evaluation? No current guidelines or standards of practice for heart disease call for doctors to assess depression. That's unacceptable. It should be standard practice for physicians to screen all patients with known coronary disease for current depressive symptoms and for past histories of depressive disorders, about once a year. Patients at high risk for developing coronary disease should also be screened for depression. Screening begins with just two questions (see Appendix D, "Assessment of Depression"), and a nurse or aide can screen people with current symptoms in five minutes. Of course, screening guidelines by themselves don't improve practice, but they provide a starting point and a standard of care. You and I can't address this problem, but the Agency for Healthcare Research and Quality can. It should revise its guidelines on unstable angina, heart failure, and cardiac rehabilitation to include specific guidelines for screening for and treating depression.[4]

3. Evaluate Depression in Cardiac Care Centers

Once guidelines for screening have been established and disseminated, the most efficient way to improve rates of recognition of depression in patients with heart disease is to evaluate depression in places where lots of people with heart disease can be found, namely, all large cardiac care centers. This means that the medical directors of coronary care units in hospitals, cardiac rehabilitation centers, and large cardiology practices should provide as part of standard cardiac care brief screening for current depressive symptoms, a review of past episodes of depression, and a review of the patient's family history of depression. Nurses and physician assistants can be trained in a half-day session to do this screening and provide standard patient education on depression and heart disease.

Screening for depression is more likely to be done, and to lead to good outcomes, if a mental health specialist is available onsite to consult and help initiate treatment planning for the patients who have depression around the time of a serious cardiac event, such as heart attack or unstable angina or angioplasty. During this period of three to six months, depression exerts its most pernicious effects on the heart, outranking most of the other common predictors of poor outcomes after a heart attack.[5] Often in busy cardiac centers the contact between the cardiologist and the patient is limited to a procedure or a single appointment during a medical crisis. With a collaborating mental health specialist available in the same center, the benefits of depression screening can translate immediately into coordinated treatment plans for both depression and the heart disease.

4. Evaluate Heart Disease in Mental Health Centers

Medical directors of mental health centers should hire primary care clinicians to provide selected primary care services in the mental health center, including evaluations for heart disease. Most chronically mentally ill people get poor medical care for a variety of reasons, including poverty, stigma, difficulty negotiating medical care, and difficulty maintaining chronic illness regimens. But their need for good medical care is urgent because the most common severe mental illnesses (depression, bipolar disorder, and schizophrenia) are also associated with higher than normal rates of smoking, obesity, diabetes, and heart disease. Mental illness is bad for the body, just as physical illness taxes the mind. And some psychiatric medications may make the medical illnesses worse. The fact that certain antidepressant and antipsychotic medications contribute to weight gain and diabetes, as we saw in Chapter 8, sharpens the argument for bringing primary care clinicians into mental health centers, where patients can see them conveniently and where collaboration among clinicians is easy.[6]

5. Educate the Public

Current public education about depression and heart disease is haphazard and inadequate. The websites of the two most influential organizations for public education about heart disease in the United States, the American Heart Association and the National Heart, Lung, and Blood Institute, have posted nothing on depression and heart disease in their public education sections. That sends the wrong message: Depression does not matter if you have heart disease. The National Institute of Mental Health has done only slightly better by posting on its website a two-page summary on depression and heart disease.[7]

In spite of the numerous self-help books on depression and an even larger number on heart disease, the first book published on the interaction of these two common disorders appeared in 2006, *The Heart-Mind Connection*, by Windsor Ting and Gregory Fricchione, a heart surgeon and a psychiatrist. In a broad look at heart disease and mental health, this book discusses eight "emotional conspirators" that aggravate heart disease: depression, anxiety, anger and hostility, social isolation, chronic life stresses, acute life stresses, panic attacks, and daily or seasonal rhythms. Each chapter provides practical suggestions on how to treat these conditions in the context of heart disease.

Meanwhile, with increasing frequency we read in newspapers and on the Web about studies that link depression and heart disease, some of them good and some not so good. With each new study the opportunities for confusion multiply. Until the leading public education organizations speak out about the evidence on depression and heart disease, it will be hard for the general public to know how to interpret the publicity about these studies and to figure out what to do. A public education campaign on depression and heart disease, jointly sponsored by the American Heart Association and the American Psychiatric Association, would begin to correct this problem.

6. Focus a Federal Research Initiative

The public health dimensions of depression and heart disease described in Chapter 2 justify establishing a federal research initiative over the next five to ten years focused on answering the key remaining questions about depression as a risk factor for coronary disease, heart disease as a risk factor for depression, and clinical trials and services research to evaluate the most effective methods for treating comorbid depression and heart disease. With new noninvasive imaging techniques for studying the functional and structural changes in the brain and the heart during the course of illness, we can now study these two disorders at a level of detail that has never before been possible. The most suitable partners for such an initiative are the National Heart, Lung, and Blood Institute (NHLBI) and the National Institute of Mental Health (NIMH). NHLBI has established a model for such a collaborative initiative in its current ACCORD study of the effect of several treatments of diabetes on coronary disease outcomes.[8] A similar joining of resources from NHLBI and NIMH to study the interaction of these two illnesses should guide the design of a project on depression and coronary disease. Without such leadership and ownership at the top, the public health problem of depression and heart disease will continue to bounce around without an advocate and without substantial funding for a coherent research strategy.

Some of these structural and procedural changes in the systems with which we treat people with depression and heart disease can be implemented by the individual patient or clinician. Others require organizational directives or policy changes. Some cost little and save a lot. Others require an investment of money and personnel. We need studies of the cost-effectiveness of these clinical innovations.[9] However, these changes are all justified as sound, evidence-based efforts to reduce the enormous suffering and costs of unrecognized depression, unrecognized heart disease, and inadequate treatment of both. Most of us—patients and clinicians—are not in a position to implement these system changes, but we're all in a position to advocate for them.

Outside the Membrane: What We Don't Know

The scientific process grows around a particular subject like an amoeba wrapping investigative pseudopods around new bits of the outside world, taking these bits in, swelling its membrane as it grows, incorporating and commanding larger and larger portions of its knowable universe. Science is all about the restless membrane of the leading questions, the creative tension between what we know and what we don't know. This book offers snapshots of the current state of this membrane surrounding what we know about depression and heart disease. It's an effort to make it possible that we patients, we doctors, and we policy makers on the local and national level all share the same knowledge and the same appreciation for what we still need to learn.

We now know, for example, that depression increases our risk for developing and dying from coronary disease. Even mild depressive symptoms increase death rates. And the more severe our depression, the higher our cardiac risk. The risk lasts a long time, more than fifteen years, according to one study. But we do not yet know whether one type of depression contributes more risk than another, or how long the depression has to last to contribute to risk. We need answers to this set of questions in order to efficiently identify who among the depressed are most at risk for heart disease and who should get the most intense treatments. As patients, we want the answers to these questions to guide our choice of treatments.

Though we know that depression is a risk factor for coronary disease, we do not yet know if it's a *major* risk factor, that is, whether depression substantially adds to the risk incurred by the six traditional major cardiac risk factors. We know that depression aggravates four of the six major risk factors, but as Figure 7.4 shows, the relative importance of depression for any person's heart disease depends on the number and severity of at least ten other factors. The scientific evidence reviewed in Chapters 2 through 6 now argues persuasively that depression matters and that depression should be considered by doctors, patients, and the American Heart Association as among the important possible contributors to the risk for coronary disease. This is even more true for women than for men, since women are twice as likely to suffer from depression and, once women develop heart disease, they tend to get less treatment and do worse than men do. But we need to understand more quantitatively how adding depression to the equation improves our ability to estimate a person's risk for heart disease, as well as our ability to treat that person.

This effort to understand the role of depression in heart disease is part of a larger effort to develop better ways of estimating risk for heart disease, such as studies of C-reactive protein and the concept of vulnerable plaque. Experts continue to debate whether we should focus on better management of the established major risk factors or search for a more predictive set of risk factors.[10]

We know a number of possible mechanisms which link depression and heart disease. Some of these behavioral and neuroendocrine mechanisms explain how depression contributes to the gradual onset of heart disease. Others better explain the later sudden cardiac event. For most people, multiple mechanisms appear likely to influence the long course of heart disease. But all these plausible mechanisms of depression's effect on heart disease remain to be proven at the level of understanding that we now have for the mechanisms of smoking and cholesterol. And we're just beginning to understand how heart disease triggers depression. We do not yet know which mechanisms play the dominant roles at which phases of the depressive or cardiac illness. That is likely to be a difficult process to study, but the better we understand these mechanisms, the more precisely we can design treatments that target them.

We know that some treatments of depression in people with heart disease are both safe and effective. We know that treating heart disease effectively can reduce depressive symptoms in some people. We can break the cycle in many ways. But, though we have ample suggestive evidence that treating depression in people with heart disease is good for their hearts, we do not yet have rigorous proof that effective depression treatment reduces the risk for the onset or progression of coronary disease. To answer that question we need several large, rigorous, randomized, and controlled clinical trials. So far, only one has been done. We need these studies because every year in this country more than ninety thousand people die at least partly as a result of depression after heart attacks, and it's likely that a substantial proportion of them could be saved with effective treatment of the depression.[11]

I believe that it's both possible and compellingly necessary for people outside the membrane of research on depression and heart disease to understand the complexities of the relationship between these two conditions. These fascinating complexities defy a single easy solution or treatment, but they also point the way to many possible approaches. I want you to leave this book with an appreciation for how understanding this complex story shows us how much we can do to improve the way we treat these conditions. I tell this story not only because of that little bone I now see growing in my heart, not only because of the moving stories of the people I work with, but also because of all the other stories, both personal and scientific, about how the troubled mind works through the brain to trouble the body. And how the body troubles the mind. Think of addictions and cancer, schizophrenia and obesity, depression and diabetes. There's a bigger lesson to learn. We're beginning to make sense of these links between the mind and the body. Making sense of depression and heart disease gives us a good start.

APPENDIXES

Appendix A. Diagnostic Criteria for Major Depressive Episode (from *DSM IV-TR*)

A. At least one of the following three abnormal moods which significantly interfered with the person's life:
   1. Abnormal depressed mood most of the day, nearly every day, for at least 2 weeks.
   2. Abnormal loss of all interest and pleasure most of the day, nearly every day, for at least 2 weeks.
   3. If 18 or younger, abnormal irritable mood most of the day, nearly every day, for at least 2 weeks.

B. At least five of the following symptoms have been present during the same 2 week depressed period.
   1. Abnormal depressed mood (or irritable mood if a child or adolescent) [as defined in criterion A].
   2. Abnormal loss of all interest and pleasure [as defined in criterion A2].

3. Appetite or weight disturbance, either:
Abnormal weight loss (when not dieting) or decrease in appetite.
Abnormal weight gain or increase in appetite.
4. Sleep disturbance, either abnormal insomnia or abnormal hypersomnia.
5. Activity disturbance, either abnormal agitation or abnormal slowing (observable by others).
6. Abnormal fatigue or loss of energy.
7. Abnormal self-reproach or inappropriate guilt.
8. Abnormal poor concentration or indecisiveness.
9. Abnormal morbid thoughts of death (not just fear of dying) or suicide.

C. The symptoms are not due to a mood-incongruent psychosis.

D. There has never been a manic episode, a mixed episode, or a hypomanic episode.

E. The symptoms are not due to physical illness, alcohol, medication, or street drugs. The symptoms are not due to normal bereavement.

Appendix B. Charting the Course of Depression

When charting the course of a depressive illness, keep it simple by identifying the severity based on mild, moderate, or severe symptoms. Along the X-axis runs time, sometimes in years, sometimes in days or months, depending on how long a period you are considering. More elaborate charts include arrows along the time line for stressful events, as well as notes. You may also track treatments above the curves to match patterns in treatments to changes in course.

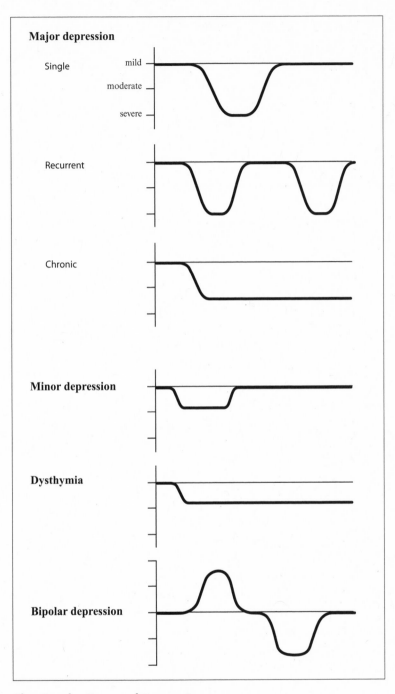

Charting the Course of Depression

Appendix C. Types of Depression

Much of the research on depression and heart disease has focused on lists of "depressive symptoms." The common lists vary from two to sixty items and include a wide range of emotional, cognitive, and physical symptoms reported by people with various types and severity of depression. Questionnaires that collect information on these symptoms measure how many symptoms a person has, as well as the frequency, duration, or intensity of the symptom. In general, the more symptoms you have, the more depressed you are. But by themselves symptoms are not enough to make a diagnosis of a depressive disorder.

The first diagnostic distinction divides large from small, serious from not so serious, major from minor depression. The diagnostic category most often studied in relation to heart disease is major depression. A major depressive episode provides the reference point around which the other depressive disorders are defined. A person meets the essential criteria for a major depressive episode if he or she (a) reports at least five of nine possible symptoms or signs of depression most of the days for at least two weeks (see criterion B under "Diagnostic Criteria for a Major Depressive Episode," in the American Psychiatric Association's *Diagnostic and Statistical Manual*); (b) reports impaired mental, social, or physical functioning as a result of these symptoms; and (c) does not have another medical or psychiatric condition which causes these symptoms.

The current distinctions among the types of depression depend on their different courses. A single major depressive episode suffices to make the diagnosis of major depressive disorder, single episode. After two episodes the diagnosis shifts to recurrent major depressive disorder, but most people with recurrent depression experience more than two episodes. In the National Comorbidity Survey, detailed in Kessler (1997), the average number of episodes reported by those with recurrent depression was more than ten. Between episodes, people with recurrent depression regain their normal functioning, but that is not true for people with chronic major depression, which describes a course of depression that lasts at least two years without full recovery. Chronic depression often persists for decades, and it's not rare to hear people with chronic depression say, "I've been depressed all my life."

Minor depression refers to a less severe disorder in which the person reports a few symptoms, usually two to four but not five or more, nearly every day for at least two weeks. Dysthymia, or chronic minor depression, refers to a course of minor depression that lasts at least two years without full recovery. Both minor depression and dysthymia raise the likelihood of developing major depression and cause significant impairment at work. Though the studies of depression and heart disease have focused less on minor than on major depression, even mild symptoms predict worse outcomes for heart disease than do no depressive symptoms.

Bipolar depression refers to a depressive episode that occurs in a person who has had at least one episode of mania. Gregory Hemingway had bipolar depression; so did his father and grandfather, in all likelihood. Bipolar disorder, also known as manic-depressive illness, inflicts the extremes of mood swings, including long periods of depression. The more common type of depression is sometimes called unipolar depression to distinguish it from bipolar depression. Bipolar depression may include simultaneous symptoms of depression and mania, such as racing thoughts or grandiosity simultaneous with suicidal despair, making it particularly difficult to diagnose and treat. Whereas major depression occurs in 8–10 percent of the general population in a given year, bipolar disorder occurs in just 1–2 percent, so bipolar depression is both less common than major depression and more complicated to manage.

The term mood disorder due to a general medical condition applies to the depression that accompanies a physical illness—for example, hypothyroidism—and resolves through treatment of that condition. Depression following a heart attack or a coronary artery bypass graft operation may be a major depression due to coronary disease, particularly if it occurs in a person with no previous history of depression and resolves with the resolution of the cardiac symptoms. Other types of depression include substance-induced mood disorder, which applies to the depression that occurs only during or following drug or alcohol abuse, such as a cocaine or alcohol binge.

Another pathway to depression follows a demanding or overwhelming event, such as a natural disaster, a betrayal, or the loss of a precious person. People who experience depressive symptoms and impaired functioning after such events, but improve within weeks, are said to have had an adjustment disorder with depressed mood. Bereavement is a common form of adjustment disorder with depressed mood. In the aftermath of these events it can be tough to tell if this depressed response will resolve on its own or will develop into a persistent major depression requiring more intensive treatment.

Finer distinctions for each of these disorders come in the form of "specifiers," which further identify key features of the disorder, such as "postpartum," or "with a seasonal pattern," or "with psychotic features." These specifiers sometimes play an important role in selecting treatments, such as light therapy for people with seasonal patterns or antipsychotic medication for people with psychotic features.

Do all these terms and distinctions matter? Why not toss them all, just call everybody depressed, and hand out the Prozac? Though there's some merit to this simplification, several crucial dimensions of depression, such as severity and duration, disappear in that simpler scenario, making it harder for the people who most need the help to get effective treatment. Effective and efficient treatment of any disorder depends on assessing the severity and duration of the disorder and understanding the factors that influence the severity and duration. In addition, some types of depression require specific kinds of treatment or imply a worse prognosis. For example, major and minor depression generally respond to the same kinds of medication and psychotherapy treatments, but bipolar depression often requires a combination of a mood-stabilizing medication, such as lithium, and an antidepressant, rather than an antidepressant alone. And recurrent depression requires longer treatment—from years to the rest of their lives for many people—as well as a focus on relapse prevention through psychotherapy, compared to briefer treatment (a few months) for simple depression or an adjustment disorder. Recurrent and chronic depression resemble heart disease in that, once contracted, the condition remains and requires varying levels of treatment for life, depending on how complicated or severe the condition is.

Appendix D. Assessment of Depression

The assessment of depression ideally begins with the patient's self-assessment. In addition to common intuition, several self-assessment or screening measures for depression can be found at *webmd.com* or *intelihealth.com*.

The standard of care in mental health circles, as well as primary care, for the assessment of depression begins with a careful history of the symptoms and the course of the depression. Two questions are usually enough to screen for depression:

1. Have you ever felt down, depressed, or hopeless for several weeks?
2. Have you ever lost interest or pleasure in doing things for several weeks?

Yes to either question should prompt further inquiry. Discussion of possible contributing or coexisting psychiatric and physical illnesses is also standard. An efficient initial depression history in a primary care setting may take two to fifteen minutes, depending on how complicated the history is. Good assessments of depression also include a medical history and a physical exam and some basic laboratory evaluations, when appropriate, to evaluate the possible contributions of such conditions as heart disease, infection, anemia, diabetes, high blood pressure, and hypothyroidism. A careful family history of depression and other psychiatric disorders may raise or lower the estimate of risk for depression. More expensive tests, such as a brain scan, may be justified in people with first episodes of severe depression, focal neurologic signs, unusual symptoms, or complex disorders. Quantitative symptom monitoring with a self-report measure of depression should be a standard part of most depression assessments.

Measures

In addition to the good judgment of the clinician, three types of measures of depression can help identify a depressive disorder: self-report questionnaires designed to detect and quantify depression symptoms; structured diagnostic interviews administered by a clinician; and biological markers such as sleep electroencephalograms (recorded brain waves), a hormone challenge test called the dexamethasone suppression test, and, most recently, certain brain scans, such as functional magnetic resonance imaging (MRI), in specially designed research studies. For a variety of reasons, none of the biological markers has so far gained acceptance for common clinical use, and this failure to define depression in biological terms that are clinically useful has hampered the study and treatment of depression.

So for now clinical practice relies almost exclusively on the clinician's judgment of the depression history and the medical data to make a diagnosis, sometimes supplemented by a self-report measure of symptoms of depression. Structured diagnostic interviews represent the best standard method for identifying a mental disorder in research settings, but they require too much time (thirty to ninety minutes to cover the major mental disorders) and training to be practical for most clinicians in busy practice settings. The best self-report measure for depression in primary care settings and cardiologists' offices, where most heart disease is treated, is the PHQ-9.

This measure is convenient and useful for both the patient and the clinician. The PHQ-9 does not include all factors that are necessary to consider before making a final diagnosis, such as what other medical or psychiatric disorders the person has, and it does not ask about past depressions, but it identifies and quantifies the severity of the key current symptoms over the previous two weeks, and it estimates the degree of impairment in the final question at the bottom. The PHQ-9 is organized according to the *DSM IV* definition of a major depressive episode, and it works well as both a self-report questionnaire and a guide for a quick interview about depression.

Scoring and interpreting the PHQ-9 is easy and can be done by the patient or the clinician. Add the numbers circled for items a–i to get a total score of 0–27. In general, 0–4 is normal, 5–9 suggests mild depression, 10–14 suggests moderate depression, and 15 or greater suggests severe depression. Most people with scores of 10 and over have major depression, that is, they score 2 or 3 on at least five of the nine a–i items, one of which is on a or b. (Because even "several days" of thoughts of suicide or hurting oneself can be a serious sign, item i counts as one of the five even if only scored 1.)

The PHQ-9 is the best aid for the primary care clinician to diagnose and monitor depression because it is free, short, easy to understand and score, and faithful to standard diagnostic criteria. It introduces a quantitative measure of severity, and, when repeated in the same person over time, the PHQ-9 provides consistency to our often intuitive and sometimes capricious methods of assessing the course of depression and its treatment.

PHQ Depression Checklist (PHQ-9)

Over the *last 2 weeks*, how often have you been bothered by any of the following problems?	Not at all	Several days	More than half the days	Nearly every day
Little interest or pleasure in doing things	0	1	2	3
Feeling down, depressed, or hopeless	0	1	2	3
Trouble falling or staying asleep, or sleeping too much .	0	1	2	3
Feeling tired or having little energy	0	1	2	3
Poor appetite or overeating.	0	1	2	3
Feeling bad about yourself—or that you are a failure or have let yourself or your family down	0	1	2	3
Trouble concentrating on things, such as reading the newspaper or watching television	0	1	2	3
Moving or speaking so slowly that other people could have noticed? Or the opposite—being so fidgety or restless that you have been moving around a lot more than usual.	0	1	2	3
Thoughts that you would be better off dead or of hurting yourself in some way.	0	1	2	3

(For office coding: Total Score _____ = ___ + ___ + ___)

If you checked off *any* problems, how *difficult* have these problems made it for you to do your work, take care of things at home, or get along with other people?

Not difficult at all   Somewhat difficult   Very difficult   Extremely difficult

---

Source: From the Primary Care Evaluation of Mental Disorders Patient Health Questionnaire (PRIME-MD PHQ). The PHQ was developed by Drs. Robert L. Spitzer, Janet B. W. Williams, Kurt Kroenke, and colleagues. For research information, contact Dr. Spitzer at rls8@columbia.edu. Printed by permission of Pfizer Inc.

Appendix E. Types of Heart Disease

A brief look at the differences among the types of heart disease will set the framework for focusing on the types that are related to the pathologic process of atherosclerosis: hypertension, coronary disease, stroke, and congestive heart failure. The types of heart disease that develop apart from atherosclerosis, such as congenital heart disease, rheumatic heart disease, and various infections of the heart, are relatively less common and not as likely to be affected by depression, so they serve this discussion mainly as points of contrast.

Atherosclerosis is both a common companion to the normal aging process of the cardiovascular system and, when excessive, a pathologic process commonly known as hardening of the arteries. That is, it is possible to identify the early stages of atherosclerosis in the vessel walls of normal children, and all adults show some evidence of the process, which increases with age. But the normal process accelerates in the presence of several of the traditional risk factors for coronary disease, which are, more precisely speaking, risk factors for atherosclerosis anywhere in the circulatory system: high LDL cholesterol, high blood pressure, smoking, diabetes, obesity, and physical inactivity.

Atherosclerosis develops throughout the cardiovascular system and contributes to several types of disease: hypertension, coronary disease, stroke, and congestive heart failure. It is rare to find advanced atherosclerosis in the vessels of the heart but not in the brain, and vice versa. The process contributes to disease when it affects the flow of blood in small arteries, usually by narrowing the diameter of the artery (in coronary arteries, narrowing by more than half qualifies as coronary disease) or by weakening the arterial wall, leading to aneurysms, leaking of blood, or full rupture.

Several of the steps in the formation of arterial plaques suggest links to depression or points where depression may hasten the transition from normal aging to pathologic hardening of the arteries. Figure 6.3, The Birth of a Plaque, shows several aspects of the atherosclerotic plaque. Note first the three layers of the vessel wall. The inner layer is a sheath of endothelial cells that controls both the diameter of the vessel and what filters through the sheath to nourish the tissues. Plaques build up between the endothelial cells and the middle layer or muscle layer of the arterial wall, eventually bulging in toward the lumen, narrowing the area of blood flow. Plaques are especially prone to develop where endothelial cells are torn or damaged. High blood pressure and sudden shifts in blood pressure increase the shear stress on the endothelial cells, especially where arteries divide into smaller branches. Depression, by contributing to blood pressure hyperreactivity during stress, may contribute to plaque formation at these sites.

When oxygen can't flow freely from the coronary arteries into the pumping heart's muscle fibers, the fibers respond with pain signals, also called anginal chest pain. In advanced atherosclerosis, large and penetrating plaques can also weaken the muscle wall of the artery, leading to bulging outward and sometimes to ruptured aneurysms.

Plaques are a form of damage to the inner arterial wall, and damage anywhere attracts blood clots, usually small and transient clots. But if the clotting mechanism is too active, making it easier than usual to form clots, or if the plaque peels away from the arterial wall, the flow in the artery may suddenly be corked, leading to a heart attack and injury to the muscle fibers downstream from the clot. Because depression increases our tendency to form clots by causing platelets to become more sticky, these clots attached to plaques may be another way that depression contributes to the progression of coronary disease.[1]

Hypertension, or high blood pressure, is often the doorway to heart disease, a person's first cardiovascular problem and often one that leads to other problems. Hypertension may precede atherosclerosis or follow it; often the two contribute to each other over many years. Several blood-pressure readings on separate days above 140/90 millimeters of mercury suffice to earn the average adult a diagnosis of high blood pressure, which simply means that the tension in the artery walls is higher than optimal. The long-term consequences of sustained high blood pressure include less efficient delivery of oxygen to the organs and more frequent wear and tear on the arterial vessel walls. Hypertension is the bread and butter of primary care, and all but the most complicated cases get treated by primary care physicians.

The majority of the fifty million Americans, one of every four U.S. adults, who have high blood pressure have no known cause for the condition. Atherosclerosis is just one of many factors that contribute to high blood pressure, but more often than not high blood pressure precedes by many years the clinical signs of atherosclerosis. Age, obesity, smoking, alcohol, and, in genetically susceptible people, high-salt diets also contribute to high blood pressure. Some types of kidney disease cause the retention of too much fluid, more than the cardiovascular system can accommodate. Rare hormonal abnormalities can also raise blood pressure.

Blood pressure normally behaves in elastic fashion, accommodating rapidly to wide ranges of demands by as much as doubling or halving its resting state values within seconds if necessary. Like a simple water balloon, the elasticity of our cardiovascular system drops as the resting blood pressure rises. Stress the system far enough, and it loses its resilience. The National Blood Pressure Education Program of the National Institutes of Public Health's Public Health Service (NIH Publication 93–1088 [1993]) sets the range for mild high blood pressure for most people at 140/90–159/99. Moderate range is 160/100–179/109. Severe range, any pressure over 180/110, often constitutes an emergency when it is a new finding, particularly if accompanied by symptoms of fatigue, headache, visual changes, chest pain, nausea, dizziness, or other signs of distress.

Most of us with mild to moderate high blood pressure don't know we have it. Only at the highest blood pressures do we feel headaches, fatigue, or visual changes. The American Heart Association has dubbed hypertension "the silent killer," drawing attention to its lack of symptoms and its influential role in strokes and heart attacks.

Coronary disease includes injury or dysfunction in any of the coronary arteries that surround the heart and feed oxygen to its muscle fibers. (The term "coronary disease" is roughly synonymous with "coronary artery disease," "atherosclerotic heart disease," "ischemic heart disease," and "coronary heart disease," but it carries the advantage of conveying the idea in two words instead of three.) Most often, atherosclerosis in the coronary artery walls is the process that results in coronary disease, but it is also possible for coronary arteries that are relatively free of atherosclerosis to develop injury or dysfunction from, for example, spasm from high doses of cocaine or nicotine. Repeated episodes of severe hypertension can damage vessel walls, or a clot that broke off an infected aortic valve can flow into the coronary artery. These other forms of coronary disease are relatively rare, but they sometimes explain the peculiar occurrence of heart attacks in a young pro athlete or a person with no traditional risk factors for atherosclerosis.

A good doctor can often diagnose coronary disease from the patient's story alone. More precise measurements of the severity of coronary disease come from the electrocardiogram, exercise stress testing, coronary angiograms, and new forms of imaging, such as CT and MRI images. Severity is defined in several ways:

1. The percent of narrowing of the inner diameter of a coronary vessel during coronary angiography, which shoots pictures of dye flowing from a catheter in the aorta into the coronary vessels and out. More than 50 percent narrowing of the diameter of any artery qualifies as coronary disease.
2. The number of coronary arteries with more than 50 percent narrowing
3. The effect of exercise on blood flow to the heart muscle as measured by the electrocardiogram or a scan of the heart.

A stroke, the brain's equivalent of a heart attack, follows when a loss of blood supply to or the rupture of a blood vessel in an area of the brain results in death of brain tissue and loss of function, such as a drooping left cheek or difficulty talking. Strokes afflict about one million adults in the United States every year, most of them over sixty-five, killing about 150,000, which makes stroke the third-most-common cause of death. Hypertension is the dominant contributing factor in about half of all strokes, whereas coronary disease contributes to just over 10 percent of strokes.[2] Most people who suffer strokes have some degree of atherosclerosis of the cerebral arteries, which impairs the circulation to the brain. Any of these conditions can set the stage for the development of the stroke by one of two mechanisms. Either the artery in the brain narrows suddenly, shutting off circulation beyond the point of narrowing, or a fragile artery ruptures, leaking blood around the rupture site and damaging it, instead of delivering it to the tissues beyond.

Strokes range in severity from the unnoticeable and insignificant (which are increasingly common with aging) to the lethal. The effects of strokes may be transient, lasting as briefly as a few days, or permanent and irreversible. More transient changes in brain function are often called transient ischemic attacks, or TIAs, because their effects don't persist for more than a few hours, but for most people TIAs warn of the high risk of a stroke with lasting effects.

Hardening of the arteries of the brain usually is a marker for hardening of the arteries elsewhere, such as in the legs or the abdomen, a condition called peripheral artery disease. Impaired circulation to the legs causes cramps when walking and is relieved by rest. Some people with particularly severe peripheral artery disease and leg cramping require bypass surgery in the abdomen or legs, similar to the bypass heart surgery that relieves coronary ischemia.

Congestive heart failure is a condition that develops when the pumping capacity of the heart weakens so much that blood fails to flow efficiently through the lungs and out to the rest of the organs. The slower-flowing blood becomes congested in the lungs and the rest of the body, leaking fluid into the tissues and causing fatigue, shortness of breath, and swelling in the feet. Any disease process that contributes to persistent weakening of the heart muscle may cause congestive heart failure. High blood pressure and atherosclerosis of the coronary arteries, which lead to gradual weakening of the heart muscle through gradual decreases in blood flow or sudden heart attacks, are the most common causes of congestive heart failure in the United States. About half the five million adults in the United States with heart failure have coronary disease as the underlying disorder that weakens the left ventricle. The rest develop heart failure from diseases of the heart valves, infections of the heart, or toxins, such as alcohol.

It's useful to think of the atherosclerotic heart diseases on a continuum of time, beginning with hypertension developing quietly and early in adult life, followed by coronary disease in the fifties and sixties, followed by stroke or congestive heart failure. Because better detection and treatment means that fewer people with coronary disease die from it now, more survive to develop congestive heart failure. Between 1970 and 2000 the number of people hospitalized in the United States with congestive heart failure more than tripled.

Rheumatic heart disease, currently affecting about 1.5 million people in the United States but more common in many developing countries, is a disease of the valves of the heart. It develops years after a childhood streptococcal infection, usually an infection as benign as a strep throat. Most people with a sore strep throat never know they have it because it's an inconvenience to get tested for it and it feels like other more common viral sore throats. Only about 3 percent of those who get strep throat later develop rheumatic fever, and a small proportion of them develop rheumatic heart disease.

Rheumatic heart disease is a poorly understood type of reaction in which the process of fighting the strep infection triggers the inflammation in the rims of the valves of the heart, causing them to leak or narrow. A heart murmur may be the first indication that there's anything wrong. Treatment of severe rheumatic heart disease often requires surgically replacing the damaged valve.

Congenital heart disease includes all problems of the heart that are present at birth. Though some are lethal, many are correctable by surgery, and all are relatively rare. The most common of the correctable problems include holes in the walls of the heart that divide one chamber from the other, atrial or ventricular septal defects. Valves may be malformed, or the vessels leading to or from the heart may be misshapen or misconnected, disrupting the normal flow of blood through the heart. Early detection and surgical correction allow for normal or nearly normal cardiac function in the best of situations. However, none of these rare congenital heart defects puts these children at greater risk in adult life for the more common heart diseases, except congestive heart failure.

Appendix F. Assessment of Heart Disease

Because the different types of heart disease require different specific tests to establish the diagnoses, no single approach applies to all types of heart disease. However, a few essential principles help to distinguish a rigorous assessment of heart disease from a sloppy one.

First, make sure your doctor provides you not just with a diagnosis, but with a complete diagnosis. That is, don't settle for a label like "heart failure" or "aortic valve disease." You and your doctor should also talk about (a) causes; (b) the anatomy affected; (c) the physiology, or how certain organs are impaired; and (d) the extent of your disability, or what your illness prevents you from doing on a daily basis.

Second, know the essential parts of a comprehensive evaluation for heart disease. In general, evaluations consist of seven methods: (1) a careful history of your symptoms; (2) a physical examination; (3) an electrocardiogram; (4) a chest X-ray; (5) noninvasive imaging studies of your heart, like an echocardiogram, or a stress test; (6) sometimes invasive imaging studies, like a cardiac catheterization study; and (7) blood tests, such as cholesterol or cardiac enzymes. Not all are necessary for all forms of heart disease.

A good assessment should consider how your heart functions both at rest and when challenged by exercise or mental stress. These evaluations can be done well by most good primary care clinicians. Cardiologists may be necessary for the assessment when other illnesses, either medical or psychiatric, complicate the picture.

Appendix G. Resources for Treatment of Depression and Stress

For guidelines on current standards for good treatment, go to *www.webmd. com*, look under Disease and Conditions, and find under *D* the Depression Health Center; a short review of Basic Treatment Options includes links to related topics. For guidelines on the treatment of anxiety and stress, look under Disease and Conditions and find Anxiety/Panic, and find Stress.

Also see the website of the National Alliance for Mental Illness at *www.nami.org*. On the home page under Welcome! click on Depression and scroll down to How Is Depression Treated. Below this section is a list of related articles.

Appendix H. Resources for Treatment of Heart Disease

For guidelines on current standards for the treatment of the various forms of heart disease, go to *www.webmd.com* and click on Diseases and Conditions. Find *H* and Heart Disease, then click on How Is It Treated? and find the Treatment Overview for coronary artery disease, for example. Also use the alphabetical index to see related sections, such as Angina, Heart Attack, Heart Failure, or Hypertension.

Also go to the American Heart Association's site at *www.american heart.org*. Under Diseases and Conditions click on Heart Attack and find Surgery and Other Treatments. For example, under Cardiac Medications, a table summarizes medication types, names, and uses.

Appendix I. Summary of a Course of Cognitive Therapy in a Fifty-One-Year-Old Man with Depression and Coronary Disease

AB, who until fifty-one had never had a problem with depression, considered himself in pretty good health. As a father of two daughters, fifteen and ten, and a husband of twenty-five years, he worked hard at his job as an industrial design expert in a large corporation, where he had done well enough to consider early retirement at fifty-five. He loved his work, "but there's just too much of it and the stress is constant," he said. Five years earlier, at forty-six, he had first learned he had an arrhythmia called atrial fibrillation, but a single medication had treated it well, and he was not worried about his heart.

Then for a few weeks he had stretches of trouble catching his breath, followed by sudden chest pain that forced him to the hospital, where he learned that he had had a heart attack and that his arrhythmia had worsened. Part of his treatment including implanting a defibrillator in his heart to prevent sudden death. When the defibrillator "fired" on his first day home, he felt he'd been "kicked in the chest." Over the next two months his energy and mood remained low, and he couldn't concentrate. He worried he wouldn't be able to return to work. "What's wrong with me? I'll never feel good again," he said to himself repeatedly.

When he began meeting with IC two months after the heart attack as part of a study of cognitive therapy for depression in people with heart disease, AB believed he was "weak, helpless, and worthless." He also believed, "If I'm unproductive or inefficient, I'm worthless," and "I'll get worse and won't be able to raise my kids." Both his grandfathers had had heart disease, and one died at fifty-five.

During the first of fourteen weekly sessions of therapy, AB scored eighteen on the Beck Depression Inventory (BDI), a self-report measure, suggesting moderate severity of symptoms, and he was given a diagnosis of major depression, based on his history. His goals included increasing his activity level, improving his emotional relationships with others, increasing communication, and learning to enjoy life in the present.

Interventions in the early sessions focused on tracking his activities with an activity log, scheduling pleasurable activities, reading about depression and heart disease, and monitoring his mood. By session four his BDI score had improved to nine, and his activity level had increased consistently.

Using a worksheet to challenge automatic thoughts about perfectionism, he learned to change both his thinking and his behavior and to accept less than perfect performance in exchange for more rewarding relationships.

The night before session five his defibrillator fired again, jolting him out of an arrhythmia and triggering a series of negative thoughts. However, he was able to counter them and prevent himself from sinking into despair about his prospects. These thoughts kept hounding him, though, and he had trouble shutting them down or finding alternatives. As he approached returning to work, his perfectionistic thought patterns arose. AB needed IC's help challenging these threatening distortions during the sessions, using thought records and learning relaxation techniques.

By session ten, AB had managed to adjust his work into a more restful balance with leisure and family. His BDI score was seven for several weeks in a row. By session thirteen, his BDI was five, in spite of his defibrillator firing for the third time. He ended therapy at session fourteen about three months after starting, having effectively recovered from his depression without using antidepressant medications. His therapy also helped him and his family manage the complex aspects of the treatment of his heart disease.

Source: This treatment summary is based on excerpts of a report provided by Iris Csik, MSW/LCSW, at the Washington University School of Medicine. Identifying details have been altered to preserve confidentiality.

NOTES

Chapter 1. The Aching Heart

1. These and other fascinating facts about heart disease can be found on the American Heart Association website at *www.americanheart.org*. Under Publications and Resources find Statistics, then Statistical Fact Sheets, then Populations, then Men and Women. The original source of the data is the National Heart, Lung, and Blood Institute, at *www.nhlbi.nih.gov/resources*: under Reports and Scientific Documents see NHLBI Fact Book and NHLBI Morbidity and Mortality Chart Book.

2. These facts on women and heart disease come from articles by Jones (2003) and Eaker (1989), and *The Women's Heart Book* by Pashkow and Libov. Also see the *Time* cover story, April 28, 2003, "Women and Heart Disease."

3. For a good review of the effect of depression on adherence to treatment regimens, see DiMatteo (2000). For a recent report on who gets treatment for depression, see Kessler (2003).

4. This information on disability and death comes from the best epidemiologic study of illness worldwide, the World Health Organization's *Global Burden of Disease Study*, summarized in Murray (1996). Or see more recent reports at *www.hsph.harvard.edu/organizations/bdu/gbdmain.htm*.

5. Many of these facts and problems are discussed in a series of articles on depression and heart disease in the *Journal of Psychosomatic Research* 2002, vol. 53, and in *Psychosomatic Medicine* 2005, vol. 67, Supplement 1.

6. For good reviews of the evidence supporting these mechanisms linking depression and heart disease, see Carney (2002) and Christenfeld (1999).

7. Three years after my interview with her, Paula Volk spent two months in an intensive care unit during a worsening of her heart failure and eventually died with her family by her side.

8. For more on why New York City, more than any other city, increases rates of heart disease, see Christenfeld (1999).

9. The argument against looking for further risk factors for coronary disease has been spelled out by Beaglehole (2002); for the counterargument, see Marmot (2002).

Chapter 2. The Size of the Problem

1. For more on warning signs of depression, see *www.nimh.nih.gov/publicat/depression.cfm*. The clinical terms for depression are discussed in detail in Chapter 3. Major depression refers to at least five symptoms for two weeks with significant impairment, whereas minor depression refers to two to four symptoms.

2. For good reviews of the role of allostatic load in stress and illness, see McEwen (1998, 2005).

3. Though we often talk about the major risk factors for heart disease when we really mean major risk factors for coronary disease, it would be even more precise if we limited the application of these risk factors to atherosclerotic heart disease, since there are other ways that coronary arteries can become "diseased" aside from atherosclerosis. Technically, these risk factors apply to the process of atherosclerosis of the coronary arteries. But the polysyllabic term "atherosclerosis" never caught on with nonclinicians and has lost out to "coronary," which is the easier term to say.

4. These six risk factors are the "major" modifiable risk factors, the factors we can do something about. Three others—age, gender, and family history of heart disease—are just as important for prediction but not treatable. For more discussion of these risk factors, go to *www.americanheart.org* and click on Heart and Stroke Encyclopedia; under *R*, find Risk Factors and Coronary Heart Disease.

5. Data on the effectiveness of smoking cessation for reducing cardiac risk come from US Department of Health and Human Services, The Health Benefits of Smoking Cessation.

6. For a discussion of the debate on how much of the risk for coronary disease is predicted by the major risk factors, see Beaglehole (2002). And see Yusuf (2005)

7. Much of this information on the epidemiology of depression can be found in Kessler (2002).

8. Novelist William Styron wrote vividly in *Darkness Visible* about the emergence of his depression after he stopped drinking in 1985: "Alcohol was an invaluable senior partner of my intellect, besides being a friend whose ministrations I sought daily—sought also, I now see, as a means to calm the anxiety and incipient dread that I had hidden away for so long somewhere in the dungeons of my spirit" (p. 40). This phenomenon of alcohol abuse masking underlying depression, and the related self-medication hypothesis, has been described extensively in the psychiatric literature, as in the American Psychiatric Association's *DSM IV*, Goodwin and Jamison's *Manic-Depressive Illness*, and Jamison's *Touched with Fire*.

9. For more on what constitutes effective treatment of depression, see Chapter 8 and Appendix G.

10. For more information on the epidemiology of depression, go to *www.nimh. nih.gov*, find Public Information on Mental Disorders, then Depression, then Depression: The Invisible Disease. The National Comorbidity Survey (NCS), the second of two major epidemiologic studies of mental illness in the United States, continues to collect data. The website for the NCS homepage, *www.hcp.med.harvard.edu/ncs/*, summarizes the major projects of the NCS, describes the methods of the studies, lists all related publications, and provides a way to request free copies. The data on the prevalence rates of current and lifetime depression come from Kessler (1997, 2003). Two other useful articles from the NCS are Blazer (1994) and Kessler (1994).

11. The estimate of 16 million with coronary disease or heart failure includes about 13.2 million with coronary disease plus about 2.5 million who have congestive heart failure without coronary disease, because about half the 5 million with congestive heart failure also have coronary heart disease. The numbers in the right column of Table 2.2 add up to more than 71 million because most people with one of these disorders also have one or more other cardiovascular disorders. For example, most people with congestive heart failure or strokes also have had coronary disease for years before developing these conditions as complications of their coronary disease. For more information on the epidemiology of heart disease, see *www.americanheart. org/statistics* and Labarthe's *Epidemiology and Prevention of Cardiovascular Diseases*.

12. Discussions of these rates can be found in reviews by Glassman (1998), Rudisch (2003), and Freedland (2003). Dr. Glassman's antidepressant study appears in Glassman (2002). The contribution of depression to poor outcomes in people with coronary disease is comparable in predictive power to most of the common predictors of outcomes of coronary disease, such as the number of coronary arteries affected, the ejection fraction of the left ventricle, or prior history of heart attacks; see Wulsin (2004).

13. For more on Denollet's Type D Personality and its relationship to heart disease, see *Newsweek's* cover story, October 3, 2005, "Stress and Your Heart." For original scientific reports, see Denollet (1995, 1996, 2001).

Chapter 3. Converging Risks

1. Klerman and Weissman (1989) were the first to note this trend of decreasing age of onset, based on more than ten studies. Data from both of the large epidemiologic studies of mental illness in the United States, the Epidemiologic Catchment Area Study and the National Comorbidity Survey, supported this observation by Kessler (2002), depicted in Fig 3.1. The National Comorbidity Study completed its first data collection in 1992 and has continued to collect data. The data on the 1966–75 cohort were

collected after 1995 when the youngest members were at least twenty. The website *www.hcp.med.harvard.edu/ncs* summarizes the major projects of the NCS, describes the methods of the studies, lists all related publications, and offers free copies.

Similar drops in the ages of onset have occurred for substance abuse during the same period, but not for most other mental disorders. Speculations about the reasons for this pattern of rising rates of depression over the latter half of the twentieth century center on the parallel rise of substance abuse and on changes in social and family structure, such as increased rates of divorce and residential moves during this period.

2. For a review of the gender differences in depression rates across cultures, see Weissman (1996). Table 3.1 is adapted from this review.

3. For more discussion of gender differences in depression, see Kessler (2000). This gender difference certainly reflects more than an artifact of the measures of depression, or a quirk in the definition of depression, or the fact that men are generally more clumsy than women when talking about feelings. This gender difference also reflects more than the disadvantaged social position of women in many cultures. How do we understand, for example, the higher female to male ratios (3.1:1 and 3:1) in relatively emancipated Germany and Italy, compared to 1.6:1 in Lebanon and Taiwan, where women live with fewer choices and less authority? For a review of the role of sex and gender differences in depression and heart disease, see Naqvi (2005).

4. For more on inheritance of depression, see Sullivan (2000). For a fascinating review of mood disorders in families of artists, see Kay Jamison's chapter, "Genealogies of These High Mortal Miseries," in *Touched with Fire*. For a review of the current knowledge about the genetic relationship between depression and heart disease, see McCaffery (2006)

5. More information on the likelihood of future episodes of depression can be found in American Psychiatric Association's *DSM IV* and Kendler (2000).

6. For more on the effect of stress on depressive episodes, see Kendler (2000).

7. For a good study of the effect of panic disorder on the risk for coronary heart disease, see Gomez-Caminero (2005).

8. The Medical Outcomes Study by Wells (1989a) was among the first to demonstrate this additive effect of depression and heart disease.

9. A good summary of gender differences in heart disease appeared in *Time* magazine's April 28, 2003, article "Women and Heart Disease." For more on death rates for women with heart disease, see Keller (2000).

10. For a concise summary of the effects of gender on the epidemiology of depression and heart disease, see Rudisch (2003).

11. Most of this increase in mortality for women results from increases in deaths from one kind of heart disease, congestive heart failure, offsetting the declining death rates for women with coronary disease. These declining

death rates for coronary disease follow dramatic public health campaign successes in dropping the rates of smoking, high blood pressure, and high cholesterol. But meanwhile, the total number of people who have heart disease has not changed because of the dramatic rises in obesity, diabetes, and physical inactivity. We've made little progress in reducing the number of people who develop heart disease. Thanks to better treatments, we live longer with our heart disease now than our parents' generation did.

Mortality statistics on heart disease come from the American Heart Association website at *www.americanheart.org*. Under Publications and Resources, find Statistics, then Biostatistical Fact Sheets, then Populations, then Men and Women. The original source of the data is the National Heart, Lung, and Blood Institute, at *www.nhlbi.nih.gov/resources*; under Reports and Scientific Documents see NHLBI Fact Book and NHLBI Morbidity and Mortality Chart Book. Also see Labarthe's *Epidemiology and Prevention of Cardiovascular Diseases*.

12. For more on smoking, depression, and heart disease, see Kaplan (1992). Among people who enroll in smoking-cessation programs, more than twice as many report a history of major depression, compared to the general population. Of course, people who enroll in smoking-cessation programs may be the most addicted of all smokers. What about smokers who don't enroll in programs to quit? One study of 1,200 young adults in a health insurance program found that smokers reported almost three times the lifetime rate of major depression (26.7 percent) as nonsmokers (9.4 percent). Even in studies such as Covey (1998) of the general population who are not selected for participating in health-care programs, the lifetime rate of major depression among smokers is almost double that of nonsmokers.

13. Nicotine is a powerful drug, among the most addictive substances. And depression makes withdrawal from nicotine more unbearable. But even after the initial withdrawal, for smokers with a past history of depression, more trouble waits down the road. In one study by Covey (1998) of smokers who managed to quit, within three months 30 percent of those with a past history of at least two episodes of major depression developed another major depressive episode, compared to 16 percent of those with a history of a single episode and 2 percent of those with no history of depression. Thirty percent relapsed into depression within three months—it's hard to argue with that kind of punishment-and-reward system. Death by lung cancer or heart disease may pose a distant threat, but depression pounces like the wolf at the door. For more on the antidepressant effects of smoking, see Laje (2001).

14. For more on the mechanisms by which smoking contributes to heart disease, see US Department of Health and Human Services, *The Health Benefits of Smoking Cessation*.

15. For a good general review of depression and diabetes, see Musselman (2003).

For more on rates of depression in diabetes, see Anderson (2001). For more on the effect of depression on glucose control, see Lustman (2000). For more on the course of depression in diabetes, see Talbot (2000).

Whether depression leads to diabetes or diabetes leads to depression depends on the type of diabetes. Type I or insulin-dependent diabetes begins in childhood, well before the usual age of onset of depression in the late teens or early twenties. And for most people with Type I, diabetes precedes the first depression, which most often follows the onset of the diabetes within a year or two. On the other hand, Type II diabetes usually doesn't strike until the forties or fifties, well after most depression–prone people have had their first depressive episode. The two studies that have looked at depression's contribution to the risk for developing Type II diabetes have concluded that depression about doubles the risk, as in Eaton (2002).

16. For more on depression and coronary disease in diabetes, see Lustman (2000) and Clouse (2003)

17. The data supporting the effects of physical inactivity on coronary disease are reviewed in Labarthe's *Epidemiology and Prevention of Cardiovascular Diseases*.

18. In one recent study by Babyak (2000), exercise by itself was as effective as sertraline (Zoloft), a common antidepressant, in helping people recover from an episode of major depression and in preventing relapse. A recent systematic review by Tkachuk (1999) of fourteen studies of exercise as a treatment for depression found that on the whole exercise improved depression as effectively as did standard psychotherapy, but debate about the impact of exercise as a treatment for depression continues because many of the studies in this area are not scientifically rigorous; see Lawlor (2001).

19. For more on depression in childhood and obesity, see Britz (2000) and Pine (2001). For more on the relationship between obesity and depression, as well as other psychiatric disorders, see Simon (2006).

20. In a study by Hopkinson (1982) of seventy-three women who were waiting for intestinal bypass surgery for severe obesity, 28 percent of the women reported a history of major depression, almost twice the lifetime rate in the general population. And 78 percent of these women reported a syndrome of short duration (several days to a week) of depressed moods with strong cravings for sweets.

21. For more on depression as a predictor of hypertension, see Davidson (2000) and Rutledge (2002).

Chapter 4. Depression: Disease of Mind, Brain, and Body

1.   Greg Hemingway, *Papa: A Personal Memoir.* p. 8.
2.   During Ernest Hemingway's final years, Greg may not have known the details of his father's medical condition, but in *Papa* he writes with medical sophistication about the extent of his father's struggle to get control over his "nerves." In *Hemingway: The Final Years* (p. 322), Michael Reynolds, writes that at age forty-seven Ernest had severely high blood pressure. Several years before he died, a physical exam revealed that he was overweight and had a cholesterol of 428 (more than double the normal level). In addition to his infamous hard drinking and ten years of taking a synthetic testosterone, he was taking medications for "high blood pressure, nerves, liver, insomnia, eyesight, and fatigue. . . . Serpasil (to relieve anxiety, tension, and insomnia), Doriden (to tranquilize), Ritalin (to stimulate the central nervous system), Eucanil, Seconal (to get to sleep), massive doses of vitamins A and B, and other drugs for an alcohol-damaged liver." In the 1950s, before effective antidepressant medications were available, he and his doctors groped for combinations of medications that would calm his nerves. Nothing worked well for long. In fact, the reserpine he took for his blood pressure may have added to his depression. In the final years before he died, when the words would no longer come, the heart and the liver of this great writer showed the ravages of his frazzled central nervous system. His mind, his brain, and his body succumbed to depression.
3.   Reynolds, *Hemingway: The Final Years*, p. 306.
4.   Five days before his death, Gregory Hemingway was arrested for intoxication and indecent exposure. Because on that day he was cross-dressing and identified himself as a woman, he was assigned to the women's section of the Miami-Dade Detention Center. According to Schoenberg (2001), his daughter Lorian claims that he was detained without his blood pressure medication and that his sudden death on the day of his hearing resulted at least in part from his lack of cardiac medications for five days while in jail.
5.   Kathy Cronkite, the daughter of Walter Cronkite, has collected personal recollections on depression from actors, journalists, and politicians in her book *On the Edge of Darkness.* This book makes easy reading and is helpful for both the new and the experienced reader about depression. Organized thematically, it combines reports of personal experiences with comments from experts and suggestions for seeking help. Also see Kay Jamison's *Touched with Fire.*
6.   I have selected some of the more vivid quotations on depression as a disease of the mind, brain, and body from Andrew Solomon's review of the history of Western approaches to depression in *The Noonday Demon: An Atlas of Depression*, Chapter 8, "History."
7.   Hippocrates, *Hippocrates*, quoted in Solomon (2001, 286).

8. Nemeroff, 1996.

9. Galen quoted in A. Roccatagliata, *A History of Ancient Psychiatry* (see Solomon [1986, 291]).

10. Robert Burton, *The Anatomy of Melancholy*, quoted in Solomon (2001, 303).

11. H. Boerhaave, *Boerhaave's Aphorisms: Concerning the Knowledge and Cure of Diseases*, quoted in Solomon (2001, 307).

12. Kraepelin is quoted in S. Jackson, *Melancholia and Depression: From Hippocratic Times to Modern Times* (see Solomon [2001, 327]). We can forgive Kraepelin for overestimating the contribution of genes or "defective heredity" to depression. A more sound estimate comes from Sullivan (2000), who estimates that genes account for about 40 percent of the variation in depression rates.

13. In *Darkness Visible* (pp. 36–37), Styron laments the inadequacy of the word "depression":

   "When I was first aware that I had been laid low by the disease, I felt a need, among other things, to register a strong protest against the word 'depression.' Depression, most people know, used to be termed 'melancholia,' a word which appears in English as early as the year 1303 and crops up more than once in Chaucer, who in his usage seemed to be aware of its pathological nuances. 'Melancholia' would still appear to be a far more apt and evocative word for the blacker forms of the disorder, but it was usurped by a noun with a bland tonality and lacking any magisterial presence, used indifferently to describe an economic decline or a rut in the ground, a true wimp of a word for such a major illness. . . . Nevertheless, for over seventy-five years the word has slithered innocuously through the language like a slug, leaving little trace of its intrinsic malevolence and preventing, by its very insipidity, a general awareness of the horrible intensity of the disease when out of control.

   "As one who has suffered from the malady in extremis yet returned to tell the tale, I would lobby for a truly arresting designation. 'Brainstorm,' for instance, has unfortunately been preempted to describe, somewhat jocularly, intellectual inspiration. . . . The phrase 'nervous breakdown' seems to be on its way out, certainly deservedly so, owing to its insinuation of a vague spinelessness, but we still seem destined to be saddled with 'depression' until a better, sturdier name is created."

14. See the American Psychiatric Association's *DSM IV-TR*.

15. Maudsley, *The Pathology of the Mind*, quoted in Solomon (2001, 32).

16. For studies supporting this estimate of risk, see Jones (2003), Penninx (2001), and Glassman (2002).

17. This link between loss and depression formed the central theme of Freud's essay "Mourning and Melancholia," in which he proposed that depression represented the mourner's often unconscious conflict about loss, either real or perceived. Unlike mourning, depression involves loss of self-esteem, "an

extraordinary diminution in self-regard." This essay catalyzed a string of efforts by others, such as Gabbard (2000), to refine this theory about the psychodynamics of depression, eventually leading to good research on the psychology of depression. Freud proposed that our anger at the lost loved one is prohibited by our conscience and by society, so we turn the anger inward, against ourselves, to spare our attachment to the loved one at some cost to our self-love. Our unconscious mind chooses depression over rage and attachment over the integrity of our ego. The fracture line opened in our ego by depression sets up the possibility of suicide, the possibility of one part of the self taking revenge on the other. Treatment and relief from the depressive conflict, Freud suggested, came with speaking one's free associations about the ambivalent feelings and raising these feelings into consciousness—the work of psychoanalysis. Then catharsis lightens the load and the therapist's understanding loosens the grip of the conflict.

18. For more on the role of life events and losses in depression, see Kendler (2002) and Li (2002).

19. Styron, *Darkness Visible*, p. 56.

20. For more on Engel's thoughts on conservation-withdrawal, see Engel (1972).

21. Beck wrote *Cognitive Therapy of Depression* for clinicians. His student David Burns has written a more readable book for the general public, *The Feeling Good Handbook*, which is both a workbook and a lively introduction to cognitive therapy for depression.

22. Aretaeus, quoted in Roccatagliata, *A History of Ancient Psychiatry* (see Solomon [2001, 290]).

23. For more on the adaptive value of depression, see Nesse (2000).

24. See Lynch (1997). Rates of depression among women on Medicaid come in part from a 2001 report, "Depression and Low-Income Women: Challenges for TANF and Welfare-to-Work Policies and Programs," at www.researchforum.org.

25. For more on depression and disability, see Druss (2000). I recently watched helplessly for six months as one of my patients in a family practice clinic spiraled down from self-sufficiency to despair and total dependency. Linda is now thirty-three and the single mother of two boys, but at twenty, ten years before I met her, she had developed a severe depression in the context of a severe eating disorder. Depression had troubled her mother and grandmother too. A suicide attempt led to two hospitalizations and five years of intensive treatment for Linda, but by the time she was thirty she had lived about five years in fairly good control of both her depression and her eating disorder. Treatment had worked.

Two years later, after a second pregnancy by a different but equally unattached guy, who also slipped away, her depression came back with a vengeance. She began compulsively eating sweets and cleaning, abandoning her meticulous attention to her cover-girl looks. She eventually lost her job, which forced her to move in with her reluctant mother. She stopped her medications because she couldn't pay for the refills. When she couldn't pay for her visits to see me, our clinic threatened to discharge her. Her mother moved to an adjacent state. Linda moved with her. It took her two months to establish residency in the new state and two more months to get approved for Medicaid, not an uncommon problem when a depressed person must navigate a new bureaucracy in a strange city. In the meantime she groped along, taking only the cheapest of the three medications she had been prescribed, barely able to clothe and feed herself and her two boys. Occasionally, she came back to our clinic to see me, hopeless, in ratty clothes, pleading for samples of antidepressant medication and anything that would let her sleep. In less than a year she had "drifted" from self-sufficiency to destitution, hobbled by severe depression, a less than helpful family, and for multiple social reasons, loss of access to treatment. Was her depression primarily a social problem? This would not have happened in Canada's or England's national health system.

26. For more on the effect of social supports on heart disease outcomes, see J. Lynch, *The Broken Heart*, Frasure-Smith (2000), and Gallo (2003).

27. See J. Lynch, *The Language of the Heart*.

28. For more on heart rate variability and death rates, see Bigger (1992).

29. In a large longitudinal study of students at Harvard and the University of Pennsylvania between 1921 and 1950, Ralph Paffenbarger (1966) examined the college-age factors that predicted the later death by coronary disease of 590 men. This study, though not a scientifically rigorous one by today's standards, was one of the first to look at a wide range of predictors for coronary disease. The list of predictive factors included some of the now traditional risk factors (smoking, high blood pressure, obesity) plus "early parental death, absence of siblings, and nonparticipation in sports." By a similar process in the same study, Paffenbarger and colleagues examined predictors of completed suicide in 225 of these graduates. Among the most predictive factors for suicide were early parental death or loss through parental separation, and nonparticipation in sports, which was interpreted by the authors as a marker for social isolation in those days.

   These associations of coronary disease and suicide with important early losses and patterns of restricted social contact have found ample confirmation in subsequent longitudinal studies conducted with greater scientific rigor, such as Everson (1996), Frasure-Smith (2000), and Vaillant (1996).

30. Styron, *Darkness Visible*, p. 48.

31. For reviews of the fascinating research on the role of "vital exhaustion" in coronary disease and its relationship to depression, see Appels (1997) and Kop (1999).

32. For more on depression and disability, see Lecrubier (2001), Murray (1996), and Wells (1989b).
33. Cronkite, *On the Edge of Darkness*, p. 32.

Chapter 5. Depression and the Biology Window

1. For more on the work for which Kandel won the Nobel Prize, see Kandel (2001) and Kandel's *In Search of Memory*.
2. For a review of the evolutionary biology of emotions, see Melvin Konner's *The Tangled Wing*.
3. For a fascinating pictorial tour of the central nervous system, see Rita Carter's *Mapping the Mind*. For an introduction to the concept of the three brains, see Paul MacLean's *The Triune Brain and Its Role in Evolution*.
4. For a full discussion of the anatomy of emotions, see Joseph LeDoux's *The Emotional Brain*.
5. Other insults in these areas of the brain, such as tumors or surgical lesions or accidental injury, also produce the signal symptoms of depression—apathy, inattentiveness, emotional instability—but with little hope for recovery.
6. These pathways to the amygdala are described in detail in Joseph LeDoux's *The Emotional Brain*. Recently I was walking alone along a dim path in the Arizona desert late at night when I jumped to my left and yelped in an uncivilized way at a shadowy movement just a few feet off the path to my right. I froze, my heart thumped, I held my breath, and I crouched, fixing on that dark spot off the path. That was my "fast loop" reflex response in action. Nothing pretty about it—you would have laughed to see the beast in me—but my reflex forced me farther away from whatever it was and forced me to focus totally on it. My first thought was that I'd seen a cactus moving. Ridiculous, but that was as good as my brain could do at first pass. My hippocampus has few cacti in its catalogue. This one looked like nothing I'd ever seen, a knee-high cone of black needles, a miniature Christmas tree of porcupine quills. And it swayed the way cacti couldn't sway. My second thought brought up the possibility of an animal, much smaller than me, and my pathway for escape if I should need it. Within seconds (was it less?) I could straighten up and feel a nervous giggle edging out my fear. I still couldn't recognize this odd swaying cactuslike thing in the dark, but my slower thalamo-cortical loop of reason had by now snuffed out my amygdala's red alert. The next day I learned that I'd met my first desert skunk, its tail straight up over its head and its amygdala firing faster than mine.
7. For more on brain-imaging studies of depression, see Mayberg (2002a), Drevets (2002), and Kennedy (2001).

8.   The hippocampus and some parts of the cingulate cortex are overactive in the early stages of a depressive episode. Later, for brief periods, areas of the prefrontal cortex that are usually underactive in depression switch into hyperactivity, presumably in a desperate attempt to dampen the overactivity of the amygdala.

It's not simple, and it's not static, but there are some patterns that dominate. As you can imagine, with a system containing as many structures and pathways and feedback loops as this emotional brain, people vary in their patterns of brain over- and underactivity. And levels of activity shift during the course of the illness, even in the absence of treatment. Early in the course of a depressive illness, the limbic system fires too much. Later, as the limbic structures lose their structural volume (the hippocampus actually shrinks) and power, they may reduce their activity below normal levels. Think of the inert, unfeeling state that immobilizes people with depressions severe enough to make them apathetic and listless. They can't feel much emotion or drum up much mental energy. The parts of their limbic systems that once were firing without restraint now may be hardly firing at all.

Shifts on the left in the anterior cingulate have different effects than shifts on the right. People also vary in how responsive they are to treatment—some people who recover show dramatic changes in the typical areas, while others show changes in atypical areas. The variation reflects individual differences in brain structure as well as differences in types of depression and responsiveness to a given treatment.

Are the brains of depressed people smaller? No, not on the whole, but several studies, such as Schatzberg (2002), have shown shrinkage of the volume of the amygdala and the hippocampus in depressed patients, though it's not yet clear whether the smaller size preceded the depression or was caused by it. The brain can regenerate some of its parts, and recovery from depression has been associated with increases in the size of the amygdala and the hippocampus. On the other hand, some loss of brain volume in depression may be permanent, as suggested by Manji (2001). R. J. Davidson (2002) found that most of the brain regions that show persistent abnormal functioning in spite of antidepressant treatment have undergone permanent structural changes and cannot regenerate. Some people with a familial vulnerability to depression have smaller-than-average anterior cingulate regions, and this area does not increase in size with improvement in depressive symptoms, according to Drevets (1997). If only the technology had been available, what would brain scans of Gloria Wachuka before, during, and after her worst depression, or of the Hemingway family over the last century, have told us about the brain during depression? Longitudinal brain-imaging studies of depression are expensive and difficult to do well, but they are currently under way, and soon we will see the depression story unfold in the brain- imaging equivalent of a movie of the brain functioning during depression.

9. For more on Mayberg's theory of depression, see Mayberg (2002b, 2003).

10. For more on the protective and damaging effects of the stress-response system, see McEwen (1998, 2005).

11. In the 1970s Carroll and Greden and colleagues at the University of Michigan first observed that about half of hospitalized patients with major depression had abnormal stress-response systems. The negative feedback loop by which high levels of cortisol normally tell the hypothalamus to cut back on its production of CRH had failed. They found high levels of cortisol that could not be suppressed by dexamethasone, a competing hormone that lowers cortisol in normal people. After a period of high hopes in the psychiatric community that this observation could lead to the development of a biological marker for depression, Carroll (1980) showed that the marker was not specific enough for depression to provide a diagnostic test. Other conditions could also produce a positive dexamethasone-suppression test, such as obesity, medications, and mania.

12. For more on cardiovascular reactivity, see Schwartz (2003). For more on the physical manifestations of the stress-response system, see Gold (2002b).

13. For a good review of the current status of our understanding of the relationship between depression and the immune system in coronary artery disease, see Kop (2005).

14. In the 1960's the first modern effort at a biological theory for depression took the form of the catecholamine hypothesis. Based on the observation that norepinephrine, a catecholamine, was abundant inside the central nervous system as well elsewhere in the body, and that some patients with depression had low levels of metabolites of norepinephrine in their urine and in their cerebrospinal fluid, Schildkraut and colleagues, such as Siever (1985) and Schatzberg (1995), proposed that depression reflected either a depletion of these hormones in the central nervous system, the out-of-gas model, or a dysregulation of them, the broken thermostat model. It soon became clear, however, that the depletion model was too simplistic. It applied to too few patients and as studies followed patients more frequently and identified new neurotransmitters, such as serotonin and dopamine, it became clear that the levels of a single neurotransmitter or its metabolite in the blood or urine could not alone account for the changes in the patient's clinical status. Since then studies, such as Charney (1999), have shown that depression is associated with dysregulation of norepinephrine at all levels of its activity: synthesis in the nerve cell, storage at the synaptic terminal, postsynaptic receptor activity, reuptake from the synapse, and metabolism once back in the cell. The dysregulation model fits the evidence better than the depletion model and now extends to all the major neurotransmitters.

15. During the first few years of the course of depressive illnesses, stressful life events tend to trigger depressive episodes, according to Kendler (2002). One effect of persistently elevated cortisol is to reduce neurogenesis in the hippocampus, that is, cortisol shuts down the ability of the hippocampus to regenerate its neural networks, which serve emotional memory and modulation of the amygdala. Normally the nerve fibers in the hippocampus constantly prune off old fibers and regenerate new fibers to sustain lively connections between nerve cells within the hippocampus. If the hippocampus can't regenerate new fibers, it atrophies and can't do its job of modulating the amygdala as well. Then the amygdala fires away unchecked. The cortex has to work harder to contain the sudden mood shifts of the unmodulated amygdala. When we sense this kind of internal stormy weather, we automatically check in more often, a kind of internal hypervigilance. Hypervigilance generates conscious worry as well, which increases CRH secretion, and the cycle perpetuates itself.

    The evidence for structural changes in the depressed brain and for shifts in the relative levels of activity in the limbic and cortical areas is recent news, mostly emerging in the past five to ten years with the arrival of powerful brain-imaging techniques. Inside the nerve cell, the relay that began with the neurotransmitters (norepinephrine, serotonin, dopamine, etc.) carrying signals across the synapses continues beyond the receptors. Triggered by the excited postsynaptic receptors, second and third messengers (cyclic AMP and phosphodiesters) normally catalyze genes in the nucleus of certain cell types in the hippocampus and amygdala to synthesize proteins that stimulate the formation of new nerve connections. These proteins that drive the formation of these new nerve connections have fancy acronyms like BDNF (brain derived neurotrophic factor) and CREB (cyclic AMP responsive element–binding protein) and NGF (nerve growth factor). A healthy amount of traffic along these lines keeps the hippocampal cells growing and remodeling, a process called "neurogenesis." Cells that generate new connections and prune out old connections are resilient and function better.

16. For more on Duman's molecular and cellular theory of depression, see Duman (1997, 2006). For a study of hippocampal atrophy, see Sapolsky (2001). For studies linking atrophy to duration of depression, see Sheline (1999) and Strakowski (2002).

Chapter 6. The Heart Has a Brain

1. The stories in the epigraphs are drawn from newspaper clippings quoted in Engel (1971, 771–782).
2. For more on Engel's biopsychosocial model of illness, see Engel (1962).
3. For the original reports on heart attacks in war zones, see Bergovec (1992).
4. For more on acute stress cardiomyopathy, see Pavin (1997).

5. For more on this study of mental stress, see Gullette (1997).

6. For data on the frequency of mental stress–induced ischemia, see Krantz (2000) and Sheps (2002). Current debates about the clinical usefulness of mental stress testing for predicting cardiovascular disease revolve around whether abnormal responses in laboratory settings relate to responses in daily life, and whether abnormal responses at one time predict a stable trait of abnormal responses over time. For good reviews, see Linden (2003), Schwartz (2003), Jain (1995), and Krantz (1999). The Krantz study showed that rising blood pressure during mental stress tests predicted worsening of atherosclerosis better than did any of the traditional risk factors that are usually used to predict outcomes.

7. For more on inflammation in heart disease, see Libby (2002b).

8. The figure is modified from Musselman (1998, 583).

9. For more on this study of chest pain pathways, see Rosen (2000).

10. The signature pathways for pain from skin, muscle, and bone are related but noticeably different from the pathways for pain from the heart and the gut.

11. In Rosen and Camici's experiment, even well after the symptoms of chest pain died down and the dobutamine (the adrenaline-like chemical that induced the ischemia) had been cleared from the system, the thalamus continued to show activity, processing signals from the heart but not forwarding them to the cortex. This observation made the investigators wonder whether in people with silent ischemia the thalamus might be doing a similar kind of editing or "gating" of signals away from the cortex. So in the second study, they repeated the same series of scans under the same conditions but this time in people with silent ischemia, those who experienced no pain when their electrocardiograms (ECG) and echocardiograms indicated mild ischemia was occurring during dobutamine infusions. None of the patients in this group experienced chest pain during the infusions, though their ECGs changed and their heart rates and blood pressure jumped just like the first group's. Their PET scans showed the same degree of thalamic activation, but significantly less cortical activation in the anterior cingulate and prefrontal cortex.

12. For more on how depression magnifies perceptions of pain after a heart attack, see Ladwig (1999)

13. For a beautifully illustrated review of the role of inflammation in atherosclerosis, see Libby (2002a).

14. Figure 6.2 is modified from Libby (2002a, 49).

15. For more on the debate about CRP in heart disease, see Pepys (2005).

16. For more on the effect of depression on inflammation, see Danner (2003) and Kop (2002). On the effect of depression and CRP on the risk for coronary disease, see Ladwig (2005).

17. From Julius (2002, 643).

18. These associations are generally more pronounced for men than for women,

though it's not yet clear why. On the effects of high heart rates, see Julius (1998) and Palatini (1999).

19. On the effects of sympathetic overactivity on atherosclerosis, see Palatini (1999).

20. On endothelial dysfunction and a causal model of heart disease, see Schwartz (2003).

21. For more on reduced mortality after reductions in heart rate, see Palatini (1999).

22. The mechanism by which this weight gain might occur is still being debated. For more on the effects of sympathetic overactivity on obesity, see Julius (2002).

Chapter 7. The Vicious Cycle: Behavioral and Biological Links

1. The metabolic syndrome is a persistent pattern of at least three of these five conditions: insulin resistance, high serum glucose, high blood pressure, obesity, or hyperlipidemia. For more on the metabolic syndrome and its relationship to stress and heart disease, see Vitaliano (2002).

2. I have adapted the figures presented in this chapter from the models proposed in the following reviews: Alexopoulos (1997), Carney (2002), Kop (1999), Musselman (1998), Rozanski (1999), Schulz (2002), Schwartz (2003), and Sloan (1999).

3. Schulz (2002) and his colleagues at the University of Pittsburgh have summarized the five pathways by which depression leads to death.

4. Interest currently focuses on the variations in the genes that regulate the serotonin transporter. For more on the genetics of depression and heart disease, see McCaffery (2006) and Williams (2001).

5. For more on stress and the genetics of depression, see Caspi (2003).

6. For a review of exhaustion and its relationship to coronary disease, see Kop (1999).

7. Figure 7.4 omits, for the sake of pictorial simplicity, many arrows that link the listed factors, such as the link between genes and most of the factors, between obesity and inflammation, and between cholesterol and plaque formation.

8. The Framingham Heart Study is the longest-running and best-known epidemiologic study of heart disease in the United States. Details on this and four other active studies (the Jackson Heart Study, CARDIA, MESA, and ARIC) are posted on the website of the National Heart, Lung, and Blood Institute at *nhlbi.nih.gov/resources*.

9. For more on the comparative effects of various psychosocial factors on heart disease, see Frasure-Smith (2003). Denollet (1998, 2001) and others have argued that prolonged distress of any kind is the important common variable

in all studies of psychosocial risk factors for coronary disease. Rozanski (1999) makes a persuasive argument for studying how the clustering of multiple psychosocial variables affects heart disease.

10. Reducing the factors that contributed to the development of the disease is the main principle of secondary prevention, that is, preventing the progression of an established disease. Primary prevention aims to prevent that disease from developing in the first place.

11. Two years later Ms. Hock, at the urging of a lipid specialist, tried a regimen of diet, daily exercise, and medication reduction. After one year on this regimen, she has regained a normal lipid profile, a normal weight, and a stable mood on three medications, instead of five, for her depression and heart disease.

Chapter 8. Is Heart Disease Depressing?

1. For reviews of the vascular depression hypothesis, see Alexopoulos (1997, 2003).

2. For a good brain-imaging study of depression in the elderly, see Thomas (2002). Two other interesting reviews, a short one by Baldwin (2002) and a long one by Rao (2000), summarize the current status of research on the vascular depression hypothesis.

3. For a review of the cognitive effects of coronary bypass surgery, see Selnes (2006).

4. Though the evidence for this cyclical relationship is based mostly on work with depression and coronary disease, the available evidence, though less ample, summarized by Freedland (2003), also supports a cyclical relationship in depression and congestive heart failure.

5. Cousins (1989), 14.

6. Cousins (1979), 39.

7. Cousins (1983), 88.

Chapter 9. Tips for Better Care

1. For more on how vascular inflammation, as measured by CRP, adds to the risk conferred by high cholesterol, see Libby (2002b).

2. These data on angioplasty and bypass rates in depressed people come from Connerney (2001); the death rates following depression after heart attack come from, among other studies, Frasure-Smith (1995).

3. The other alternative to preventive antidepressant treatment during the period after bypass surgery or angioplasty is a plan of heightened vigilance. You can monitor your own depression symptoms every one to two weeks using a rating scale such as the PHQ-9 or the Beck Depression Inventory

(see Appendix D) and, if symptoms rise above an agreed-upon cutoff score, contact the doctor and initiate an aggressive treatment plan early. At the very least this vigilant approach will reduce the misery and costs of a prolonged full depressive episode, minimizing the chance that depression will sabotage the treatment of the heart disease. At best, this approach will improve the course of the heart disease.

4. For more on the effectiveness of cardiac rehabilitation, see Taylor (2004). For more on the frequency of cardiac rehabilitation use in the United States, see Covey (1998).

5. For more on the clinical benefits of the Cretan Mediterranean diet, see Singh (2002) and de Lorgeril (1999).

6. The studies of rates of depression in countries with varying levels of fish intake come from Mamalakis (2002) and Noaghiul (2003).

7. A summary of treatment studies of omega-3 fatty acid supplements for heart disease can be found at *www.americanheart.org* , search for Fish and Omega-3. Treatment studies of omega-3 fatty acid supplements for depression include Nemets (2002), Mischoulon (2000), and Stoll (1999).

8. For a study of vitamin intervention for stroke prevention, see Spence (2005).

9. Studies on exercise as a treatment for heart disease include Taylor (2004). Studies on exercise as a treatment for depression include Blumenthal (1999) and Babyak (2000). The evidence for exercise as a treatment for heart disease is stronger than the evidence for exercise as a treatment for depression because there have been more good heart-disease studies.

10. The American Heart Association website provides extensive tips and guides to programs on how to make exercise a part of your daily life for good effect on your heart (*www.americanheart.org*, see section on exercise and fitness in Healthy Lifestyle on the main menu).

11. For a good review of beta-blockers and their side effects, see Ko (2002). Though this and other reviews fail to find a causal link between beta-blockers and depression in large numbers of patients, these reviews do not deny the experience of the small number of patients who feel depressive symptoms as side effects of beta-blockers. In other words, though we physicians should not, as a rule, avoid using beta-blockers in people at risk for depression, we may have to modify their use in the few who respond to beta-blockers with depressive symptoms. And all beta-blockers are not the same. Because propranolol is the beta-blocker that most easily crosses from the blood into the brain, it is the one most likely to contribute to depressive symptoms if taken over a long period of time. Atenolol or timolol are least likely to cross the blood-brain barrier.

12. The assertion that SSRIs are safe and effective in coronary disease is based on the collective clinical experience with these medications over the past decade in the United States and in Europe, the current standard of practice,

and a few clinical trials, such as Glassman (2002) and ENRICHD (2003). The protective effects of SSRIs have been reported in Sauer (2001, 2003).

13. For a good review of tricyclic antidepressants in heart disease, see Roose (1994).

14. For a report on how cardiac risk factors interfere with antidepressant treatment response, see Iosifescu (2005).

15. For a good review of erectile dysfunction in depression and heart disease, see Roose (2003).

16. Another promising treatment is enhanced external counterpulsation (EECP), an effective, noninvasive procedure that requires seven weeks of thirty-five one-hour sessions, during which three pairs of pneumatic cuffs, similar to large blood-pressure cuffs, are wrapped around the calves, lower thighs, and upper thighs. The cuffs rapidly inflate and deflate in time with the cycle of the heartbeat in a way that increases blood flow to the multiple sites, including the coronary vessels, while reducing systolic blood pressure. Not only does this procedure improve cardiac function for up to five years in patients with an initial favorable response, according to Bonetti (2003), but Springer (2001) found that EECP also improves depressive symptoms.

17. For more on the Dean Ornish program, see Ornish (1996) and Dean Ornish, MD's Lifestyle Program on *www.webmd.com.*

18. For more on psychotherapy in the management of heart disease, see Allan (1998) and van Peski-Oosterbaan (1999).

19. For a good review of light therapy for depression, see Avery (2001).

20. For a good review of ECT and heart disease, see Applegate (1997).

21. For a study of the effect of pet ownership on heart-rate variability in survivors of heart attacks, see Friedmann (2003).

22. For more on herbal treatments of heart disease and the spirit, see *Chinese Herbal Medicine,* by Bensky and Gamble.

23. Half of all people in the United States who have died from heart attacks did not know that they had heart disease, according to Beaglehole (2002). Less than half of all people with hypertension get effective treatment for it (*www. americanheart.org,* click on Heart and Stroke Encyclopedia, then click on *H* and High Blood Pressure Statistics). And Kessler (2003) found that only two thirds all people with major depression in the United States get any treatment at all, with only 22 percent of those with major depression in the past year receiving "adequate" treatment.

24. In 2001 the Institute of Medicine, the most influential think tank on health policy in this country, for the first time advocated a major overhaul of the U.S. health-care system. The best summary of these recommendations is the institute's *Crossing the Quality Chasm: A New Health System for the 21st Century.*

25. The information on the incidence of coronary disease in the United States comes from Rosamond (1998).

Chapter 10. A Call for Change

1. This Institute of Medicine report, *Crossing the Quality Chasm: A New Health System for the 21st Century*, is available at www.iom.edu/reports under 2001 Reports.

2. This Institute of Medicine report, *Priority Areas for National Action: Transforming Health Care Quality*, is available at www.iom.edu/reports under 2003 Reports.

3. For more on the effectiveness of integrating mental health care into primary care, see Katon (1996), Rollman (2003), and Pincus (2003)

4. The Agency for Healthcare Research and Quality posts its guidelines on its website at www.ahrq.gov; click on Clinical Practice Guidelines. The guidelines for cardiac rehabilitation are #17 under Clinical Practice Guideline Products. Guidelines for unstable angina, #10, and for congestive heart failure, #11, are under Clinical Practice Guidelines Archives.

5. The evidence supporting this effect of depression on outcomes after heart attacks is reviewed in Chapter 2, and in Carney (2003).

6. For more on efforts to establish primary care services for the mentally ill, see Chafetz (2004) and Ohlsen (2005).

7. Searching for "depression" on the AHA website produces a list of about ten relevant articles on recent studies linking depression and heart disease. But there are more than forty good original studies on this subject and more than fifteen good reviews, few of which appear on this website. The word "depression" has not yet made it into the Heart and Stroke Encyclopedia of this website. This oversight reflects both the gap between the cultures of mental illness and physical illness and the gap between research and practice. Combine the two gaps and you see the gap between psychiatric research on depression and the medical practice of cardiac care. The AHA's section on stress is relegated to the miscellaneous part of the risk-factors section under Warnings; it is brief and vague, and it never mentions depression, the effect of psychiatric disorders on cardiac morbidity or mortality, or the use of psychotropic medications for the treatment of stress. For the NIMH website entry, see www.nimh.gov, click on Depression, then on Occurrence with Other Serious Illnesses, then Depression and Cardiovascular Disease.

8. The ACCORD Study is jointly funded by NHLBI, the institute responsible for funding studies related to heart disease, and NIDDK, the institute responsible for funding projects related to diabetes. Its main aim is to study whether tight control of diabetes reduces the risk for heart disease.

9. The few cost-effectiveness studies that have been done suggest a promising effect for depression treatments. For more on these studies, see Glassman (2003), DiMatteo (2000), and Ziegelstein (2001).

10. This debate is summarized in the series of articles by Beaglehole (2002) and Marmot (2002).

11. For more on the epidemiology supporting this estimate of the number of deaths attributable to depression after heart attacks, see Carney (2003).

Appendix E. Types of Heart Disease

1. See Musselman (1998).
2. See Labarthe, Epidemiology and Prevention of Cardiovascular Diseases.

REFERENCES

Alexopoulos G, Meyers B, Young R, Campbell S, Silbersweig D, Charlson M. Vascular depression hypothesis. *Psychosomatic Medicine* 1997; 58:113–21.

Alexopoulos G. Vascular disease, depression, and dementia. *Journal of the American Geriatric Society* 2003; 51:1178–80.

Allan R, Scheidt S. Group psychotherapy for patients with coronary heart disease. *International Journal of Group Psychotherapy* 1998; 187–214.

American Psychiatric Association. *Diagnostic and Statistical Manual of Mental Disorders [DSM IV-TR]*. 4th ed. Text Revision. Washington, DC: American Psychiatric Association; 2000.

Anderson R, Freedland K, Clouse R E, Lustman P J. The prevalence of comorbid depression in adults with diabetes: a meta-analysis. *Diabetes Care* 2001; 24:1069–78.

Appels A. Depression and coronary heart disease: observations and questions. *Journal of Psychosomatic Research* 1997; 43:443–52.

Applegate R. Diagnosis and management of ischemic heart disease in the patient scheduled to undergo electroconvulsive therapy. *Convulsive Therapy* 1997; 13:128–44.

Avery D, Eder D, Bolte M, Hellekson C, Dunner D, Vitiello M, et al. Dawn simulation and bright light in the treatment of SAD: a controlled study. *Biological Psychiatry* 2001; 50:205–16.

Babyak M, Blumenthal J, Herman S, Parinda K. Exercise treatment for major depression: maintenance of therapeutic benefit at 10 months. *Psychosomatic Medicine* 2000; 62:633–38.

Baldwin R, O'Brien J. Vascular basis of late-onset depressive disorder. *British Journal of Psychiatry* 2002; 180:157–60.

Beaglehole R, Magnus P. The search for new risk factors for coronary heart disease: occupational therapy for epidemiologists? *International Journal of Epidemiology* 2002; 31:1117–22.

Beck A T, Rush A J, Shaw B F, Emery G. *Cognitive Therapy of Depression*. New York: Guilford Press; 1978.

Bensky D, Gamble A. *Chinese Herbal Medicine*. Revised ed. Seattle: Eastland Press; 1993. Translated by Bensky D, Gamble A.

Bergovec M, Mihatov S, Prpic H, Rogan S, Batarelo V, Sjerobarski V. Acute myocardial infarction among civilians in Zagreb city area. *Lancet* 1992; 339:303.

Bigger J T, Fliess J, Steinman R. Frequency domain measures of heart period variability and mortality after myocardial infarction. *Circulation* 1992; 85:164–71.

Blazer D G, Kessler R C, McGonagle K A, Swartz M. The prevalence and distribution of major depression in a national community sample: the National Comorbidity Survey. *American Journal of Psychiatry* 1994; 151:979–86.

Blumenthal J A, Babyak M A, Moore K A, Craighead W E, Herman S, Khatri P, et al. Effects of exercise training on older patients with major depression. *Archives of Internal Medicine* 1999; 159 (19): 2349–56.

Boerhaave H. *Boerhaave's Aphorisms: Concerning the Knowledge and Cure of Diseases.* London: W Innys and C Hitch; 1742; referenced in Solomon (2001).

Bonetti P, Holmes D, Lerman A, Barsness G. Enhanced external counterpulsation for ischemic heart disease: what's behind the curtain? *Journal of the American College of Cardiology* 2003; 41:1918–25.

Britz B, Siegfried W, Ziegler A, Lamertz C. Rates of psychiatric disorders in a clinical study of adolescents with extreme obesity and in obese adolescents ascertained via population based study. *International Journal of Obesity* 2000; 24:1707–14.

Burns D D. *The Feeling Good Handbook.* New York: William Morrow; 1999.

Burton R. *Anatomy of Melancholy.* T C Faulkner; N K Kiessling; R L Blair, editors. Oxford: Clarendon Press; 1997.

Carney R, Freedland K, Miller G, Jaffe A. Depression as a risk factor for cardiac mortality and morbidity: a review of potential mechanisms. *Journal of Psychosomatic Research* 2002; 53:897–902.

Carney R M, Freedland K E. Depression, mortality, and medical morbidity in patients with coronary heart disease. *Biological Psychiatry* 2003; 54 (3): 241–47.

Carroll B J, Feinberg M, Greden J F, Haskett R, James N, Steiner M, et al. Diagnosis of endogenous depression: comparison of clinical, research, and neuroendocrine criteria. *Journal of Affective Disorders* 1980; 2:177–94.

Carter R. *Mapping the Mind.* Berkeley, Los Angeles, London: University of California Press; 1998.

Caspi A, Sugden K, Moffitt T E, Taylor A, Craig I W, Harrington H, et al. Influence of life stress on depression: moderation by a polymorphism in the 5-HTT gene. *Science* 2003; 301:386–89.

Chafetz L, Collins-Bride G M, White M. A nursing faculty practice for the severely mentally ill: merging practice with research. *Nursing Outlook* 2004; 52 (4): 209–14.

Charney D S, Nestler E J, Bunney B S. *The Neurobiology of Mental Illness.* Oxford: Oxford University Press; 1999.

Christenfeld N, Glynn L, Phillips D, Shrira I. Exposure to New York City as a risk factor for heart attack mortality. *Psychosomatic Medicine* 1999; 61:740–43.

Clouse R E, Lustman P J, Freedland K E, Griffith L S, McGill J B, Carney R M. Depression and coronary heart disease in women with diabetes. *Psychosomatic Medicine* 2003; 65 (3): 376–83.

Connerney I, Shapiro P, McLaughlin J, Bagiella E, Sloan R. Relation between depression after coronary artery bypass surgery and 12-month outcome: a prospective study. *Lancet* 2001; 358:1766–71.

Cousins N. *Anatomy of an Illness as Perceived by the Patient: Reflections on Healing and Regeneration.* New York: WW Norton; 1979.

———. *Head First: The Biology of Hope and the Healing Power of the Human Spirit.* New York: Dutton; 1989.

———. *The Healing Heart: Antidotes to Panic and Helplessness.* New York: Norton; 1983.

Covey L S, Glassman A H, Stetner F. Cigarette smoking and major depression. In: M S Gold; B Stimmel, editors. *Smoking and Illicit Drug Use.* Binghamton, N.Y.: Haworth Medical Press; 1998.

Cronkite K. *On the Edge of Darkness.* New York: Bantam Doubleday Dell; 1994.

Damasio A. *Descartes' Error: Emotion, Reason, and the Human Brain.* New York: HarperCollins; 1994.

Danner M, Kasl S, Abramson J, Vaccarino V. Association between depression and elevated c-reactive protein. *Psychosomatic Medicine* 2003; 65:347–56.

Davidson K, Jonas B, Dixon K, Markovitz J. Do depressive symptoms predict early hypertension incidence in young adults in the CARDIA study? *Archives of Internal Medicine* 2000; 160:1495–1500.

Davidson R J, Lewis D A, Alloy L B, Amaral D G, Bush G, Cohen J, et al. Neural and behavioral substrates of mood and mood regulation. *Biological Psychiatry* 2002; 52:478–502.

de Lorgeril M, Salen P, Martin J L, Monjaud I, Delaye J, Mamelle N. Mediterranean diet, traditional risk factors, and the rate of cardiovascular complications after myocardial infarction: final report of the Lyon Diet Heart Study. *Circulation* 1999; 99 (6): 779–85.

Denollet J, Sys S, Brutsaert D. Personality and mortality after myocardial infection. *Psychosomatic Medicine* 1995; 57:582–91.

Denollet J, Sys S, Stroobant N, Rombouts H, Gillebert T, Brutsaert D. Personality as independent predictor of long-term mortality in patients with coronary heart disease. *Lancet* 1996; 347:417–21.

Denollet J, Brutsaert D. Personality, disease severity, and the risk of long-term cardiac events in patients with a decreased ejection fraction after myocardial infarction. *Circulation* 1998; 97:167–73.

Denollet J. Reducing emotional distress improves prognosis in coronary heart disease. *Circulation* 2001; 104:2018–23.

DiMatteo M, Lepper H, Croghan T. Depression is a risk factor for noncompliance with medical treatment. *Archives of Internal Medicine* 2000; 160:2101–7.

Drevets W, Bogers W, Raicle M. Functional anatomical correlates of antidepressant drug treatment assessed using PET measures of regional glucose metabolism. *European Neuropsychopharmacology* 2002; 12:527–44.

Drevets W, Price J L, Simpson J, Todd R, Reich T, Vannier M, et al. Subgenual prefrontal cortex abnormalities in mood disorders. *Nature* 1997; 386:824–27.

Druss B G, Rosenheck R A, Sledge W H. Health and disability costs of depressive illness in a major US corporation. *American Journal of Psychiatry* 2000; 157:1274–78.

Duman R S, Heninger G, Nestler E J. A molecular and cellular theory of depression. *Archives of General Psychiatry* 1997; 54:597–606.

Duman R S, Monteggia L M. A neurotrophic model for stress-related mood disorders. *Biological Psychiatry* 2006; 59 (12): 1116–27.

Eaker E D. Psychosocial factors in the epidemiology of coronary heart disease in women. *Psychiatric Clinics of North America* 1989; 12 (1): 167–73.

Eaton W. Epidemiologic evidence on the comorbidity of depression and diabetes. *Journal of Psychosomatic Research* 2002; 53:903–6.

Engel G L. *Psychological Development in Health and Disease*. Philadelphia: W B Saunders; 1962.

———. Sudden and rapid death during psychological stress. *Annals of Internal Medicine* 1971; 74:771–82.

Engel G, Schmale A. Conservation-withdrawal: a primary regulatory process for organismic homeostasis. *Ciba Foundation Symposia* 1972; 8:57–75.

ENRICHD. Effects of treating depression and low perceived social support on clinical events after myocardial infarction. *Journal of the American Medical Association* 2003; 289:3106–16.

Everson S, Goldbert D, Kaplan G, Cohen R, Pukkala E, Tuomilehto J, et al. Hopelessness and risk of mortality and incidence of myocardial infarction and cancer. *Psychosomatic Medicine* 1996; 58:113–21.

Frasure-Smith N, Lesperance F, Talajic M. Depression and 18-month prognosis after myocardial infarction. *Circulation* 1995; 91:999–1005.

Frasure-Smith N, Lesperance F, Gravel G, Masson A, Juneau M, Talajic M, et al. Social support, depression, and mortality during the first year after myocardial infarction. *Circulation* 2000; 101:1919–24.

Frasure-Smith N, Lesperance F. Depression and other psychological risks following myocardial infarction. *Archives of General Psychiatry* 2003; 60:627–36.

Freedland K, Rich M, Skala J, Carney R, Davila-Roman V, Jaffe A. Prevalence of depression in hospitalized patients with congestive heart failure. *Psychosomatic Medicine* 2003; 65:119–28.

Freud S. Mourning and Melancholia. In: J Strachey, editor. *The Standard Edition* of the Complete Psychological Works of Sigmund Freud. Vol. 14. London: Hogarth Press; 1917; pp. 239–60.

Friedmann E, Thomas S A, Stein P K, Kleiger R E. Relation between pet ownership and heart rate variability in patients with healed myocardial infarcts. *American Journal of Cardiology* 2003; 91 (6): 718–21.

Gabbard G. *Psychodynamic Psychiatry in Clinical Practice.* 3rd ed. Washington, DC: American Psychiatric Press; 2000.

Gallo L, Troxel W, Kuller L, Sutton-Tyrrell K, Edmundowicz D, Matthews K. Marital status, marital quality, and atherosclerotic burden in postmenopausal women. *Psychosomatic Medicine* 2003; 65:952–62.

Glassman A, Shapiro P. Depression and the course of coronary artery disease. *American Journal of Psychiatry* 1998; 155:4–11.

Glassman A, O'Connor C, Califf R, Swedeberg K, Schwartz P, Bigger J J, et al. Sertraline treatment of major depression in patients with acute MI or unstable angina. *Journal of the American Medical Association* 2002; 288:701–9.

Glassman A, Shapiro P, Ford D, Culpepper L, Finkel M, Swenson J, et al. Cardiovascular health and depression. *Journal of Psychiatric Practice* 2003; 9:409–21.

Gold P W, Charney D. Depression: disease of mind, brain, and body. *American Journal of Psychiatry* 2002a; 159:1826.

Gold P W, Drevets W, Charney D. New insights into the role of cortisol and the glucocorticoid receptor in severe depression. *Biological Psychiatry* 2002b; 52:381–85.

Gomez-Caminero A, Blumentals W A, Russo L J, Brown R R, Castilla-Puentes R. Does panic disorder increase the risk of coronary heart disease? A cohort study of a national managed care database. *Psychosomatic Medicine* 2005; 67(5): 688–91.

Goodwin F, Jamison K. *Manic-Depressive Illness.* Oxford: Oxford University Press; 1990. pp. 151–53.

Gullette E, Blumenthal J, Babyak M, Jiang W, Waugh R, Frid D, et al. Effects of mental stress on myocardial ischemia during daily life. *Journal of the American Medical Association* 1997; 277:1521–26.

Hemingway G. *Papa: A Personal Memoir.* Boston: Houghton Mifflin; 1976.

Hippocrates. *Hippocrates.* London: William Heinemann; 1962. Translation of: W Jones; E Withington.

Hopkinson G, Bland R. Depressive syndromes in grossly obese women. *Canadian Journal of Psychiatry* 1982; 27:213–15.

Institute of Medicine. *Crossing the Quality Chasm: A New Health System for the 21st Century.* Washington, DC: National Academy of Sciences; 2001.

Iosifescu D V, Clementi-Craven N, Fraguas R, Papakostas G I, Petersen T, Alpert J E, et al. Cardiovascular risk factors may moderate pharmacological treatment effects in major depressive disorder. *Psychosomatic Medicine* 2005; 67(5): 703–6.

Jackson S. *Melancholia and Depression: From Hippocratic Times to Modern Times.* New Haven and London: Yale University Press; 1986.

Jain D, Burg M, Soufer R, Zaret B. Prognostic implication of mental stress-induced silent left ventricular dysfunction in patients with stable angina pectoris. *American Journal of Cardiology* 1995; 76:31–35.

Jamison K R. *Touched with Fire: Manic-Depressive Illness and the Artistic Temperament.* New York: Free Press; 1993.

Jones D, Bromberger J, Sutton-Tyrrell K, Matthews K. Lifetime history of depression and carotid atherosclerosis in middle-aged women. *Archives of General Psychiatry* 2003; 60:153–60.

Julius S, Palatini P, Nesbitt S D. Tachycardia: an important determinant of coronary risk in hypertension. *Journal of Hypertension* 1998; 16 (Suppl1): S9–S15.

Julius S. The association of tachycardia with obesity and elevated blood pressure. *Journal of Pediatrics* 2002; 140:643–5.

Kandel E. The molecular biology of memory storage: a dialogue between genes and synapses. *Science* 2001; 294:1030–38.

———. *In Search of Memory: The Emergence of a New Science of Mind.* New York: WW Norton; 2006.

Kaplan G, Cohen R, Wilson T, Kauhanen J, Salonen T, Salonen R. Depression amplifies the association between carotid atherosclerosis and age, hypertension, low density lipoproteins, and platelet aggregability. American Heart Association Press; 1992. (32nd Annual Conference on Cardiovascular Epidemiology, Dallas, March 19–21, 1992).

Katon W, Robinson P, VonKorff M, Lin E, Bush T, Ludman E, et al. A multifaceted intervention to improve treatment of depression in primary care. *Archives of General Psychiatry* 1996; 53:913–19.

Keller M B. Citalopram therapy for depression: a review of 10 years of European experience and data from U.S. clinical trials. *Journal of Clinical Psychiatry* 2000; 61(12): 896–908.

Kendler K S, Thornton L M, Gardner C O. Stressful life events and previous episodes in the etiology of major depression in women: an evaluation of the "kindling" hypothesis. *American Journal of Psychiatry* 2000; 157:1243–51.

Kendler K S, Sheth K, Gardner C, Prescott C. Childhood parental loss and risk for first-onset of major depression and alcohol dependence: the time-decay of risk and sex differences. *Psychological Medicine* 2002; 32:1187–94.

Kennedy S H, Evans K R, Kruger S, Mayberg H S, Meyer J H, McCann S, et al. Changes in regional brain glucose metabolism measured with positron emission tomography after paroxetine treatment of major depression. *American Journal of Psychiatry* 2001; 158:899–905.

Kessler R C. Gender differences in major depression. In: E Frank, editor. *Gender and Its Effect on Psychopathology.* Washington, DC: American Psychiatric Press; 2000.

———. Epidemiology of depression. In: I Gotlib; C Hammen, editors. *Handbook of Depression.* New York: Guilford Press; 2002; pp. 23–42.

Kessler R C, Berglund P, Demler O, Jin R, Koretz D, Merikangas K, et al. The epidemiology of major depressive disorder: results from the National Comorbidity Study Replication (NCS-R). *Journal of the American Medical Association* 2003; 289:3095–105.

Kessler R C, McGonagle K A, Zhao S, Nelson C B, Hughes M, Eshelman S, et al. Lifetime and 12-month prevalence of DSM-III-R psychiatric disorders in the United States. *Archives of General Psychiatry* 1994; 51:8–19.

Kessler R C, Zhao S, Blazer D G, Swartz M. Prevalence, correlates, and course of minor depression and major depression in the National Comorbidity Survey. *Journal of Affective Disorders* 1997; 45:19–30.

Klerman G, Weissman M. Increasing rates of depression. *Journal of the American Medical Association* 1989; 261:2229–35.

Ko D, Hebert P, Coffey C, Sedrakayan A, Jeptha C, Krumholz H. Beta-blocker therapy and symptoms of depression, fatique, and sexual dysfunction. *Journal of the American Medical Association* 2002 (288):351–57.

Konner M. *The Tangled Wing.* New York: W H Freeman; 2001.

Kop W J. Chronic and acute psychological risk factors for clinical manifestations of coronary artery disease. *Psychosomatic Medicine* 1999; 61:476–86.

Kop W J, Gottdiener J, Tangen C, Fried L, McBurnie M, Walston J, et al. Inflammation and coagulation factors in persons >65 years of age with symptoms of depression but without evidence of myocardial ischemia. *American Journal of Cardiology* 2002; 89:419–24.

Kop W J, Gottdiener J S. The role of immune system parameters in the relationship between depression and coronary artery disease. *Psychosomatic Medicine* 2005; 67 Suppl 1:S37–S41.

Krantz D S, Santiago H T, Kop W J. Prognostic value of mental stress testing in coronary artery disease. *American Journal of Cardiology* 1999; 84:1292–97.

Krantz D S, Sheps D S, Carney R M, Natelson B H. Effects of mental stress in patients with coronary artery disease: evidence and implications. *Journal of the American Medical Association* 2000; 283:1800–1802.

Labarthe D R. *Epidemiology and Prevention of Cardiovascular Diseases.* Gaithersburg, Maryland: Aspen Publishers; 1998.

Ladwig K, Roll G, Breithardt G, Borggrefe M. Extracardiac contributions to chest pain perception in patients 6 months after acute myocardial infarction. *American Heart Journal* 1999; 137 (3):528–35.

Ladwig K H, Marten-Mittag B, Lowel H, Doring A, Koenig W. C-reactive protein, depressed mood, and the prediction of coronary heart disease in initially healthy men: results from the MONICA-KORA Augsburg Cohort Study 1984–1998. *European Heart Journal* 2005; 26 (23):2537–42.

Laje R P, Berman J A, Glassman A H. Cigarette smoking and major depression. *Current Psychiatry Reports* 2001; 3:470–74.

Lawlor D A, Hopker S W. The effectiveness of exercise as an intervention in the management of depression: systematic review and meta-regression analysis of randomised controlled trials. *British Medical Journal* 2001; 322:763–67.

Lecrubier Y. The burden of depression and anxiety in general medicine. *Journal of Clinical Psychiatry* 2001; 62 Suppl 8:4–9.

LeDoux J. *The Emotional Brain: The Mysterious Underpinnings of Emotional Life.* New York: Simon & Schuster; 1996.

Li J, Hansen D, Mortensin P, Olsen J. Myocardial infarction in parents who lost a child: a nationwide prospective cohort study in Denmark. *Circulation* 2002; 106:1634–9.

Libby P. Atherosclerosis: the new view. *Scientific American* 2002a; May:47–55.

Libby P, Ridker P, Maseri A. Inflammation and atherosclerosis. *Circulation* 2002b; 105:1135–43.

Linden W, Gerin W, Davidson K. Cardiovascular reactivity: status quo and a research agenda for the new millennium. *Psychosomatic Medicine* 2003; 65 (1):5–8.

Lustman P J, Anderson R, Freedland K E, de Groot M, Carney R M, Clouse R E. Depression and glycemic control: a meta-analytic review of the literature. *Diabetes Care* 2000; 23:934–42.

Lynch J, Kaplan G, Shema S. Cumulative impact of sustained economic hardship on physical, cognitive, psychological, and social functioning. *New England Journal of Medicine* 1997; 337:1889–95.

Lynch J J. *The Broken Heart: The Medical Consequences of Loneliness.* New York: Basic Books; 1977.

———. *The Language of the Heart: The Body's Response to Human Dialogue.* New York: Basic Books; 1985.

MacLean P. *The Triune Brain and Its Role in Evolution.* New York: Plenum Press; 1990.

Mamalakis G, Tornaritis M, Kafatos A. Depression and adipose essential polyunsaturated fatty acids. *Prostaglandins Leukotrienes and Essential Fatty Acids* 2002; 67 (5):311–18.

Manji H K, Drevets W, Charney D. The cellular neurobiology of depression. *Nature Medicine* 2001; 7:541–47.

Marmot M. Commentary: occupational therapy or major challenge? *International Journal of Epidemiology* 2002; 31:1122–24.

Maudsley H. *The Pathology of the Mind.* London: Macmillan; 1895.

Mayberg H. Depression,II: Localization of psychopathology. *American Journal of Psychiatry* 2002a; 159:1979.

———. Modulating limbic-cortical circuits in depression: targets of antidepressant treatments. *Seminars in neuropsychiatry* 2002b; 7:255–68.

Mayberg H S. Positron emission tomography imaging in depression: a neural systems perspective. *Neuroimaging Clinics of North America* 2003; 13(4): 805–15.

McCaffery J M, Frasure-Smith N, Dube M P, Theroux P, Rouleau G A, Duan Q, et al. Common genetic vulnerability to depressive symptoms and coronary artery disease: a review and development of candidate genes related to inflammation and serotonin. *Psychosomatic Medicine* 2006; 68(2): 187–200.

McEwen B S. Protective and damaging effects of stress mediators. *New England Journal of Medicine* 1998; 338:171–79.

————. Stressed or stressed out: what is the difference? *Journal of Psychiatry and Neuroscience* 2005; 30(5): 315–18.

————. Glucocorticoids, depression, and mood disorders: structural remodeling in the brain. *Metabolism: Clinical and Experimental* 2005b; 54 (5 Suppl 1): 20–23.

McKhann G M, Grega M A, Borowicz L M, Jr., Baumgartner W A, Selnes O A. Stroke and encephalopathy after cardiac surgery: an update. *Stroke* 2006; 37(2): 562–71.

Mischoulon D, Fava M. Docosahexanoic acid and omega-3 fatty acids in depression. *Psychiatric Clinics of North America* 2000; 23(4): 785–94.

Murray C, Lopez A. *The Global Burden of Disease: Summary.* Cambridge, Mass.: Harvard School of Public Health; 1996.

Musselman D, Evans D, Nemeroff C. The relationship of depression to cardiovascular disease. *Archives of General Psychiatry* 1998; 55:580–92.

Musselman D L, Betan E, Larsen H, Phillips L S. Relationship of depression to diabetes types 1 and 2: epidemiology, biology, and treatment. *Biological Psychiatry* 2003; 54(3): 317–29.

Naqvi T Z, Naqvi S S, Merz C N. Gender differences in the link between depression and cardiovascular disease. *Psychosomatic Medicine* 2005; 67 Suppl 1:S15–S18.

Nemeroff CB. The corticotropin-releasing factor (CRF) hypothesis of depression: new findings and new directions. *Molecular Psychiatry* 1996; 1:336–42.

Nemets B, Stahl Z, Belmaker R H. Addition of omega-3 fatty acid to maintenance medication treatment for recurrent unipolar depressive disorder. *American Journal of Psychiatry* 2002; 159(3): 477–79.

Nesse R. Is depression an adaptation? *Archives of General Psychiatry* 2000; 57:14–20.

Noaghiul S, Hibbeln J R. Cross-national comparisons of seafood consumption and rates of bipolar disorders. *American Journal of Psychiatry* 2003; 160(12): 2222–27.

Ohlsen R, Peacock G, Smith S. Developing a service to monitor and improve physical health in people with serious mental illness. *Journal of Psychiatric and Mental Health Nursing* 2005; 12:614–19.

Ornish D. *Dr. Dean Ornish's Program for Reversing Heart Disease: The Only System*

Scientifically Proven to Reverse Heart Disease without Drugs or Surgery. New York: Ivy Books; 1996.

Paffenbarger R. Chronic disease in former college students. *American Journal of Public Health* 1966; 56:962–71.

Palatini P, Julius S. The physiological determinants and risk correlations of elevated heart rate. *American Journal of Hypertension* 1999; 12:3S-8S.

Pashkow F, Libov C. *The Women's Heart Book.* New York: Hyperion; 2001.

Pavin D, Le Breton H, Daubert C. Human stress cardiomyopathy mimicking acute myocardial syndrome. *Heart* 1997; 78:509–11.

Penninx B, Beekman A, Honig A, Deeg D, Schoevers R, van Eijk J, et al. Depression and cardiac mortality. *Archives of General Psychiatry* 2001; 58:221–27.

Pepys M B. CRP or not CRP? That is the question. *Arteriosclerosis, Thrombosis, and Vascular Biology* 2005; 25(6): 1091–94.

Pincus H A, Hough L, Houtsinger J K, Rollman B L, Frank R G. Emerging models of depression care: multi-level ("6 P") strategies. *International Journal of Methods of Psychiatric Research* 2003; 12(1): 54–63.

Pine D S, Goldstein R B, Wolk S, Weissman M. The association between childhood depression and adulthood body mass index. *Pediatrics* 2001; 107:1049–56.

Prochaska J, Norcross J, DiClimente C. *Changing for Good.* New York: Avon Books; 1994.

Rao R. Cerebrovascular disease and late life depression: an age-old association revisited. *International Journal of Geriatric Psychiatry* 2000; 15:410–33.

Reynolds M. *Hemingway: The Final Years.* New York: W W Norton; 1999.

Roccatagliata G. *A History of Ancient Psychiatry.* New York: Greenwood Press; 1986.

Rollman B L, Herbeck Belnap B, Reynolds C F, Schulberg H C, Shear M K. A contemporary protocol to assist primary care physicians in the treatment of panic and generalized anxiety disorders. *General Hospital Psychiatry* 2003; 25(2): 74–82.

Roose S, Glassman A, Attia E, Woodring S. Comparative efficacy of selective serotonin reuptake inhibitors and tricyclics in the treatment of melancholia. *American Journal of Psychiatry* 1994; 151:1735–39.

Roose S. Depression: links with ischemic heart disease and erectile dysfunction. *Journal of Clinical Psychiatry* 2003; 64 Suppl 10:26–30.

Rosamond W, Chambliss L, Folsom A, Cooper L, Conwill D, Clegg L, et al. Trends in the incidence of myocardial infarction and in mortality due to coronary heart disease, 1987 to 1994. *New England Journal of Medicine* 1998; 339:861–67.

Rosen S D, Camici P G. The brain-heart axis in the perception of cardiac pain: the elusive link between ischaemia and pain. *Annals of Medicine* 2000; 32:350–64.

Rozanski A, Blumenthal J, Kaplan J. Impact of psychological factors on the pathogenesis of cardiovascular disease and implications for therapy. *Circulation* 1999; 99:2192–217.

Rudisch B, Nemeroff C. Epidemiology of comorbid coronary artery disease and depression. *Biological Psychiatry* 2003; 54:227–40.

Rutledge T, Hogan B. A quantitative review of prospective evidence linking psychological factors with hypertension development. *Psychosomatic Medicine* 2002; 64:758–66.

Sapolsky R. Depression, antidepressants, and the shrinking hippocampus. *Proceedings of the National Academy of Science USA* 2001; 98:12320–22.

Sauer W, Berlin J, Kimmel S. Selective serotonin reuptake inhibitors and myocardial infarction. *Circulation* 2001; 104:1894–98.

———. Effect of antidepressants and their relative affinity for the serotonin transporter on the risk of myocardial infarction. *Circulation* 2003; 108:32–36.

Schatzberg A. Brain imaging in affective disorders: more questions about causes versus effects. *American Journal of Psychiatry* 2002; 159:1807–8.

Schatzberg A F, Schildkraut J J. Recent studies on norepinephrine systems in mood disorders. In: F Bloom; D J Kupfer, editors. *Psychopharmacology: The Fourth Generation of Progress.* New York: Raven; 1995.

Schoenberg N. *The Son Also Falls.* Chicago Tribune 2001; November 19.

Schulz R, Drayer R A, Rollman B L. Depression as a risk factor for non-suicide mortality in the elderly. *Biological Psychiatry* 2002; 52:205–25.

Schwartz A R, Gerin W, Davidson K, Pickering T G, Brosschot J F, Thayer J F, et al. Toward a causal model of cardiovascular responses to stress and the development of cardiovascular disease. *Psychosomatic Medicine* 2003; 65:22–35.

Selnes O A, McKhann G M, Borowicz L M, Jr., Grega M A. Cognitive and neurobehavioral dysfunction after cardiac bypass procedures. *Neurologic Clinics* 2006; 24(1): 133–45.

Sheline Y I, Sanghavi M, Mintun M A, Gado M H. Depression duration but not age predicts hippocampal volume loss in medically healthy women with recurrent major depression. *Journal of Neuroscience* 1999; 19:5034–43.

Sheps D, McMahon R, Becker L, Carney R, Freedland K, Cohen J, et al. Mental-stress induced ischemia and all-cause mortality in patients with coronary artery disease. *Circulation* 2002; 105:1780–84.

Siever L J, Davis K L. Toward a dysregulation hypothesis of depression. *American Journal of Psychiatry* 1985; 142:1017–31.

Simon G E, Von Korff M, Saunders K, Miglioretti D L, Crane P K, van Belle G, et al. Association between obesity and psychiatric disorders in the US adult population. *Archives of General Psychiatry* 2006; 63(7): 824–30.

Singh R B, Dubnov G, Niaz M A, Ghosh S, Singh R, Rastogi S S, et al. Effect of an Indo-Mediterranean diet on progression of coronary artery disease in high risk patients (Indo-Mediterranean Diet Heart Study): a randomised single-blind trial. *Lancet* 2002; 360(9344): 1455–61.

Sloan R, Shapiro P, Bagiella E, Myers M, Gorman J. Cardiac autonomic control buffers blood pressure variability responses to challenge: a psychophysiologic model of coronary artery disease. *Psychosomatic Medicine* 1999; 61:58–68.

Solomon A. *The Noonday Demon: An Atlas of Depression.* New York: Scribner; 2001.

Spence J, Bang H, Chambless L, Stampfer M. Vitamin intervention for stroke prevention trial: an efficacy analysis. *Stroke* 2005; 36:2404–9.

Springer S, Fife A, Lawson W, Hui J, Jandorf L, Cohn P, et al. Psychosocial effects of enhanced external counterpulsation in the angina patient: a second study. *Psychosomatics* 2001; 42:124–32.

Stoll A, Severus W, Freeman M. Omega-3 fatty acids in bipolar disorder: a preliminary double-blind, placebo-controlled trial of eicosapentanoic acid in bipolar depression. *Archives of General Psychiatry* 1999; 56:407–12.

Strakowski S M, DelBello M P, Zimmerman M E, Getz G E, Ret J, Shear P, et al. Ventricular and periventricular structural volumes in first- versus multiple-episode bipolar disorder. *American Journal of Psychiatry* 2002; 159:1841–47.

Styron W. *Darkness Visible: A Memoir of Madness.* New York: Vintage Books; 1990.

Sullivan P F, Neale M C, Kendler K S. Genetic epidemiology of major depression: review and meta-analysis. *American Journal of Psychiatry* 2000; 157:1552–62.

Talbot F, Nouwen A. A review of the relationship between depression and diabetes in adults. *Diabetes Care* 2000; 23:1556–62.

Taylor R, Brown A, Ebrahim S, Jolliffe J, Noorani H, Rees K, et al. Exercise-based rehabilitation for patients with coronary heart disease: systematic review and meta-analysis of randomized controlled trials. *American Journal of Medicine* 2004; 116:714–16.

Thom T, Haase N, Rosamond W, Howard V J, Rumsfeld J, Manolio T, et al. Heart disease and stroke statistics—2006 update: a report from the American Heart Association Statistics Committee and Stroke Statistics Subcommittee. *Circulation* 2006; 113: e85–151.

Thomas A, O'Brien J, Davis S, Ballard C, Barber R, Kleria R, et al. Ischemic basis for deep white matter hyperintensities in major depression. *Archives of General Psychiatry* 2002; 59:785–92.

Ting W, Fricchione G. *The Heart-Mind Connection: How Emotions Contribute to Heart Disease and What to Do about It.* New York: McGraw-Hill; 2006.

Tkachuk G, Martin G. Exercise therapy for patients with psychiatric disorders: research and clinical implications. *Professional Psychology: Research and Practice* 1999; 30:275–82.

US Department of Health and Human Services. *The Health Benefits of Smoking*

Cessation. Rockville, Md.: US Department of Health and Human Services; 1990.

Vaillant G, Orav J, Meyer S, Vaillant L, Roston D. Late-life consequences of affective spectrum disorder. *Inter Psychogeriatrics* 1996; 8:13–31.

van Peski-Oosterbaan A, Spinhoven P, van Rood Y, van der Does J, Bruschke A, Rooijmans H. Cognitive-behavioral therapy for noncardiac chest pain: a randomized trial. *American Journal of Medicine* 1999; 106:424–29.

Vitaliano P, Scanlan J, Zhang J, Savage M, Hirsch I, Siegler I. A path model of chronic stress, the metabolic syndrome, and coronary heart disease. *Psychosomatic Medicine* 2002; 64:418–35.

Weissman M M, Bland R C, Canino G J, et al. Cross-national epidemiology of major depression and bipolar disorder. *Journal of the American Medical Association* 1996; 276:293–99.

Wells K, Golding J, Burnam M. Affective, substance abuse, and anxiety disorders in persons with arthritis, diabetes, heart disease, high blood pressure, or chronic lung conditions. *General Hospital Psychiatry* 1989a; 11:320–27.

Wells K, Stewart A, Hays R, Burnam A, Rogers W, Daniels M, et al. The functioning and well-being of depressed patients. *Journal of the American Medical Association* 1989b; 262:914–19.

Williams R, Marchuk D, Kishore K, Barefoot J, Grichnik K, Helms M, et al. Central nervous system function and cardiovascular responses. *Psychosomatic Medicine* 2001; 63:300–305.

Wulsin L R. Is depression a major risk factor for coronary disease? A systematic review of the epidemiologic evidence. *Harvard Review of Psychiatry* 2004; 12:79–93.

Yusuf S, Hawken S, Ounpuu S, Dans T, Avezum A, Lanas F, et al. Effect of potentially modifiable risk factors associated with myocardial infarction in 52 countries (the INTERHEART study): case control study. *Lancet* 2004; 364:937–52.

Ziegelstein R. Depression in patients recovering from myocardial infarction. *Journal of the American Medical Association* 2001; 161:1621–27.

INDEX

Page numbers in *italics* indicate clinical tips; those in **bold** indicate figures or tables.